COMMON
FOOT PROBLEMS
IN PRIMARY
CARE

COMMON FOOT PROBLEMS IN PRIMARY CARE

Richard B. Birrer, M.D., FAAFP, FACP
Associate Professor of Medicine
Cornell University Medical College
Associate Professor of Family Medicine
State University of New York Health Science
   Center at Brooklyn
Attending, Department of Family Practice
   and Community Medicine
Catholic Medical Center of Brooklyn and Queens
Jamaica, New York

Michael P. DellaCorte, D.P.M., FACFS
Associate Clinical Professor, External Faculty
New York College of Podiatric Medicine
Diplomate, American Board of Podiatric Surgery
Co-ordinator of Podiatric Research and Publication
Assistant Director of Podiatric Medical Education
Catholic Medical Center of Brooklyn and Queens
Jamaica, New York

Patrick J. Grisafi, D.P.M., FACFS
Associate Clinical Professor, External Faculty
New York College of Podiatric Medicine
Diplomate, American Board of Podiatric Surgery
Chief, Department of Podiatric Surgery
Director of Podiatric Medical Education
Catholic Medical Center of Brooklyn and Queens
Jamaica, New York

HANLEY & BELFUS, INC./Philadelphia
MOSBY-YEAR BOOK, INC./St. Louis • Baltimore • Boston • Chicago • London
Philadelphia • Sydney • Toronto

Publisher: HANLEY & BELFUS, INC.
210 S. 13th Street
Philadelphia, PA 19107
(215) 546-7293

North American and worldwide sales and distribution:

MOSBY-YEAR BOOK, INC.
11830 Westline Industrial Drive
St. Louis, MO 63146

In Canada: THE C.V. MOSBY COMPANY, LTD.
5240 Finch Avenue East
Unit 1
Scarborough, Ontario M1S 5A2
Canada

Common Foot Problems in Primary Care   ISBN 1-56053-050-2

Library of Congress Catalog Card Number 92-70040

Last digit is the print number: 9 8 7 6 5 4 3 2 1

CONTENTS

CONTRIBUTORS

Richard B. Birrer, MD, FAAFP, FACP
Associate Professor of Medicine
Cornell University Medical College
Associate Professor of Family Medicine
State University of New York Health Science
    Center at Brooklyn
Attending, Department of Family Practice
    and Community Medicine
Catholic Medical Center of Brooklyn and Queens
Jamaica, New York

Karen A. Borsos, DPM
Resident
Department of Podiatry
St. Joseph's Hospital, A Division of Catholic
    Medical Center of Brooklyn and Queens
Jamaica, New York

William F. Buffone, DPM
Chief Resident
Department of Podiatry
St. Josephs's Hospital, A Division of Catholic
    Medical Center of Brooklyn and Queens
Jamaica, New York

Gus Constantouris, DPM, RPh
Resident
Department of Podiatry
St. Joseph's Hospital, A Division of Catholic
    Medical Center of Brooklyn and Queens
Jamaica, New York

Michael P. DellaCorte, DPM, FACFS
Associate Clinical Professor, External Faculty
New York College of Podiatric Medicine
Diplomate, American Board of Podiatric Surgery
Co-ordinator of Podiatric Research
    and Publication
Assistant Director of Podiatric Medical Education
Catholic Medical Center of Brooklyn and Queens
Jamaica, New York

Patrick J. Grisafi, DPM, FACFS
Associate Clinical Professor, External Faculty
New York College of Podiatric Medicine
Diplomate, American Board of Podiatric Surgery
Chief, Department of Podiatric Surgery
Director of Podiatric Medical Education
Catholic Medical Center of Brooklyn and Queens
Jamaica, New York

Daniel L. Picard, MD, FACS
Assistant Professor of Surgery
Cornell University Medical College
Director of Surgery and Associate Program Director
Department of Surgery
St. Joseph's Hospital, A Division of Catholic
    Medical Center of Brooklyn and Queens
Jamaica, New York

Stuart Plotkin, DPM
Diplomate, American Board of Podiatric Orthopedics
Attending Podiatrist, Department of Podiatry
St. Joseph's Hospital, A Division of Catholic
    Medical Center of Brooklyn and Queens
Jamaica, New York

Paul V. Porcelli, DPM
Resident, Department of Podiatry
St. Joseph's Hospital, A Division of Catholic
    Medical Center of Brooklyn and Queens
Jamaica, New York

Caren B. Schumer, DPM
Attending Podiatrist, Department of Podiatry
St. Joseph's Hospital, A Division of Catholic
    Medical Center of Brooklyn and Queens
Jamaica, New York

John Tsouris, DPM
Resident, Department of Podiatry
St. Joseph's Hospital, A Division of Catholic
    Medical Center of Brooklyn and Queens
Jamaica, New York

Acknowledgments

The authors give special thanks to Cary Aloise, Janet Christensen,
Denise DellaCorte, BSN, Jason Dennis, Lester Dennis, DPM, Richard
Leichter, Miriam Ligowski, Steven Mehl, DPM, Sharon Taylor,
Katherine Ward, and Maryanne Zielinski.

DEDICATION

To Herbert Rausher, D.P.M. (in memoriam), and the Kings County Hospital Center Podiatry Group.

Richard B. Birrer

To my wife, Denise, for her patience and understanding throughout this long project.

Michael P. DellaCorte

PREFACE

To him whose feet hurt, everything hurts.

Socrates

"My feet are killing me" and "Oh, my aching feet" are two common American complaints. According to a recent Gallup poll, nearly 75% of individuals over 18 years of age complained that their feet hurt. An incredible 62% of them believed that their feet were supposed to hurt! Women were afflicted more than men. At least one third of women attributed their foot pain to uncomfortable shoes; 45% wore those shoes because they looked good. Twenty percent of these same women would not relinquish style for comfort. In 1986, at least $300 million was spent on insoles, corn remedies, bunion removers, foot powders, and other over-the-counter foot care products. Such problems do not exist in the "noncivilized" populations of the world where shoes are not worn! Ironically, the majority of people consider the foot the ugliest part of their body.

From a medical perspective, the foot is similarly neglected through both omission and commission. How many of us examine the foot as carefully as we examine other parts of the body? Although virtually all health care providers are knowledgeable in examination of the foot, less than 50% perform such examination on a regular basis. Worse still, the foot is overlooked in whole or in part some 66% of the time in the management of patients with diabetes or peripheral vascular disease. Lack of formal clinical rotations in podiatry and the traditional separation of the medical and podiatric specialties are major reasons why medical practitioners overlook the foot care of their patients. The foot can no longer be regarded as an unsophisticated static appendage joining the leg to the ground. Rather the foot is a dynamically functional, marvelously designed structure that in many ways is even more intricately constructed and specially modified than the hand. Indeed the human foot is engineered not only to last a lifetime but also to withstand an incredible amount (115,000 miles) of wear along the way.

This text is specifically designed for primary care practitioners, who see the majority of patients with healthy and diseased feet. The comprehensive nature of the primary care specialties (internists, family practitioners, nurse practitioners, physician's assistants, and pediatricians) mandates more than a cursory concern for patients' feet. It is the goal of this text to guide practitioners in the care of healthy and diseased feet, assist them in maintaining preventive vigilance, and, above all, improve the partnership they share with these patients. Lastly, the value of this book transcends basic and clinical sciences and treatment guidelines. The specialties of medicine and podiatry are uniquely blended so that each can share in the wisdom and experience of the other.

Richard B. Birrer, M.D.
Michael P. DellaCorte, D.P.M.
Patrick J. Grisafi, D.P.M.

Chapter 1

ANATOMY

Richard B. Birrer, M.D.

OSTEOLOGY

The foot is composed of 26 bones and 55 articulations and is responsible for transmitting the ground reactive force to the body during standing, ambulation, and other activities (Fig. 1). The bones of the foot can be conveniently divided into three regions: forefoot, midfoot, and rearfoot. The forefoot is represented by the 14 bones of the toes and five metatarsals. The midfoot consists of the three cuneiform bones, the cuboid, and the navicular. Finally, the rearfoot, or the greater tarsus, is composed of the talus and the calcaneus. The foot contains two arches: longitudinal (midpart) and transverse (forepart). The transverse arch forms the convexity of the dorsum of the foot. The tarsal and tarsometatarsal articulations constitute the longitudinal arch, which is maintained primarily by the plantar ligaments and aponeurosis. An individual's feet are as individual as he or she is; in fact, each foot on an individual is distinctive. Often, it is these minor variations, in each foot, that alter the mechanics of the feet and cause subsequent sequelae.

Like the hand, the phalanges of the foot are similar in number and distribution, although they are somewhat shorter and broader than their counterparts in the hand. Proximally the five metatarsals articulate with both the lesser tarsus and themselves through broad concavities, whereas distally they taper to join the phalanges through convex heads. The first metatarsal is the shortest and strongest; it contains plantar articulation for the two sesamoid bones (tibial and fibular) located in the tendons of the flexor hallucis brevis. The second metatarsal is the longest and the least

mobile of the metatarsals and serves as the anatomical keystone for abduction and adduction of the foot. The fifth metatarsal is noted for its lateral prominence (styloid process), which serves as the insertion site of the tendon of the peroneus brevis. The styloid area is often avulsed during acute inversion injuries of the foot (Jones fracture).

Distally, the three cuneiform bones (medial, intermediate, and lateral) assist in the formation of the transverse arch. The cuneiforms with the cuboid and their articulations to the metatarsals form Lisfranc's joint. The midtarsal joint is formed by the articulations of the navicular to the talus and the calcaneus to the cuboid.

The largest tarsal bone, the calcaneus (os calcis), serves three basic functions. Most of the body's weight, which is transmitted through the talus, is borne by the calcaneus and, because of its high percentage of cancellous bone, is the site of compression fractures. Posteriorly, the calcaneus completes the longitudinal arch. The calcaneus, through its articulation with the talus, joins the foot to the leg. The articulation forms a canal or groove termed the sinus tarsi. Finally, the posterior third of the calcaneus serves as the insertion point for the tendoachillis, thus providing an effective lever for calf muscle insertion. The anterior third of the calcaneus involves articulation with the cuboid bone (the calcaneal-cuboid joint or the midtarsal joint of Chopart) and a middle facet, termed the sustentaculum tali, for attachment with the talus.

The attachment of the foot to the leg occurs through the talus (astragalus). Medially and laterally, the talus articulates with the tibial and fibular malleoli, forming, with the talar

1

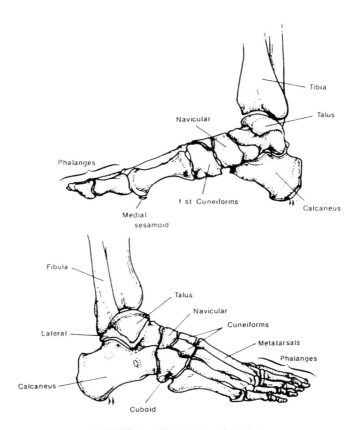

FIGURE 1. The bones of the foot.

trochlea, the uniaxial ankle joint. The anterior portion of the talar trochlea is wider than the posterior portion and curves slightly, thus providing inherent stability during dorsiflexion but instability in plantar flexion. Both are the principal motions of the ankle joint. The fibrous joint capsule provides additional support, especially medially and laterally. The talus has no muscular attachments and, combined with high-pressure forces per square inch, is susceptible to vascular damage during trauma. Fractures of the talus, therefore, are frequently associated with avascular necrosis.

There are a number of sesamoids and accessory bones variably present in the foot. The sesamoids are usually present within tendons juxtaposed to articulations and are often incompletely ossified (e.g., contain cartilage, fibrous tissue, and bone). The tibial (medial) and fibular (lateral) sesamoids of the flexor hallucis brevis are always present plantar to the first metatarsal head. The lateral one is usually single, but the medial one may be bipartite, tripartite, or quadripartite. It is

important to ascertain that any multipartite sesamoid is present bilaterally before fracture is considered. Other locations where sesamoids may be found are under the heads of the four lateral metatarsals or in the tendons of the tibialis anterior, tibialis posterior, or peroneus longus. Between the ages of 10 and 20, accessory bones appear in the foot. Common examples include an os trigonum at the posterior plantar surface of the talus, an accessory navicular bone (os tibiale externum) located at the medial border, and ossicles at the base of the fifth metatarsal (os vesalianum), intermetatarsal, interphalangeal, and intercuneiform areas.

SYNDESMOLOGY

The medial collateral ligament of the ankle joint or deltoid ligament has both superficial and deep components (Fig. 2). Superficially, the ligament consists of tibionavicular, tibiocalcaneal, and posterior tibiotalar components.

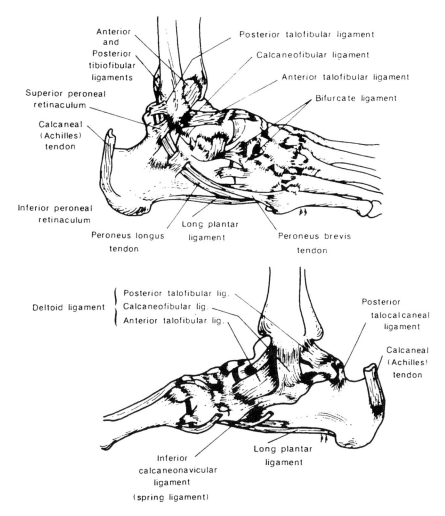

FIGURE 2. The medial and lateral ligaments of the ankle.

The anterior middle component also stabilizes the subtalar joint. The deep portion of the deltoid ligament is the anterior tibiotalar ligament, which is responsible for stabilizing the medial malleolus and talus. Laterally, the ligamentous structure is not as sturdy, consisting of three ligaments: the anterior talofibular, calcaneofibular, and posterior talofibular ligament. The lateral collateral ligament is commonly torn with inversion sprains, whereas the deltoid is rarely torn.

The subtalar joint (talocalcaneal) is surrounded by a thin, nonsupportive joint capsule. Stability in the joint is maintained essentially by four sturdy ligaments: the interosseous, medial collateral, talocalcaneal, and cervical ligaments. The interosseous, medial collateral, and talocalcaneal ligaments prevent excessive eversion, whereas the cervical and lateral collateral ligaments inhibit inversion.

The spring ligament (inferior calcaneonavicular ligament) serves to articulate the navicular bone with the sustentaculum tali of the calcaneus. The ligaments of the calcaneocuboid joint include the plantar ligaments and a portion of the bifurcate ligament. The plantar ligaments help maintain the longitudinal arch. The bifurcate ligament can be injured during forced inversion.

The plantar aponeurosis consists of a very strong fibrous central portion and a small, thinner medial and lateral section. Each is oriented longitudinally on the plantar aspect of the foot. The central portion runs from the medial calcaneal tuberosity and inserts distally, with the superficial portion attaching the skin to the pads of the toes and a deeper portion blending with flexor tendon sheaths. The medial and lateral components of the plantar aponeurosis provide vertical intermusculature septa for the plantar musculature. This aponeurosis is analogous to the one in the hand.

Three important ankle retinacula bind the leg tendons as they enter the foot. The extensor retinacula consists of two portions: superior and inferior. Continuous with the deep leg fascia and joint (the anterior, lateral, and medial malleolus), the superior extensor retinaculum serves to contain the tendons of the extensor digitorum longus, extensor hallucis longus, tibialis anterior, and the peroneus tertius. The Y-shaped inferior retinaculum consists of upper and lower bands, and it runs from the lateral calcaneus to the medial tibial malleolus and plantar aponeurosis, thus preventing "bow stringing" of the dorsal tendon in the conjunction with the superior retinaculum. Coursing between the distal fibula and the lateral calcaneus are the peroneal retinacula, which firmly secure the peroneus longus and brevis tendon behind the fibular malleolus. Medially, the flexor retinaculum extends from the calcaneus to the tibial malleolus and provides a firm support structure for the neurovascular bundle, flexor digitorum longus, flexor hallucis longus, and tibialis posterior.

MYOLOGY

The muscles of the foot can be divided into extrinsic and intrinsic components (Figs. 3 and 4). The extrinsic muscles consist of the muscles of the anterior, posterior, and lateral compartments of the leg. The posterior compartment consists of the posteriorly located flexors of the foot (i.e., gastrocnemius, plantaris, and soleus). The gastrocnemius and plantaris arise from the femur, whereas the soleus originates from the posterior surface of the proximal fibula and tibia. The three muscles collectively constitute the triceps surae and are innervated by branches of the tibial nerve.

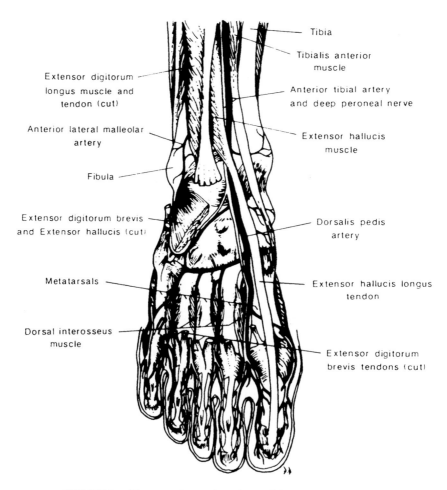

FIGURE 3. The muscles and tendons of the dorsum of the foot.

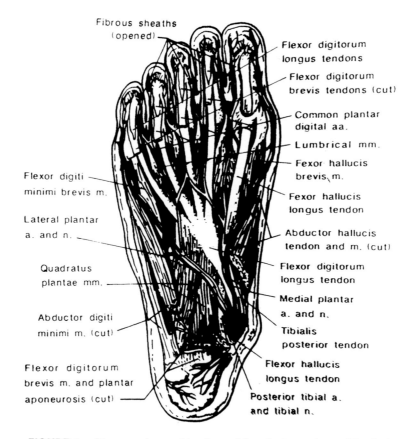

FIGURE 4. The muscles and tendons of the plantar surface of the foot.

They form the tendocalcaneus (Achilles) as they merge to insert into the posterior calcaneus. The Achilles is the largest and the strongest tendon in the human body. It consists of fibers derived not only from the two heads of the gastrocnemius but also from the soleus and plantaris. The remaining extrinsic flexors course behind the medial malleolus. They are the tibialis posterior, flexor digitorum longus, and flexor hallucis longus. The tibialis posterior inserts into the navicular bone, the medial and intermediate cuneiforms, and the base of the second, third, and fourth metatarsals. The tibialis posterior maintains the longitudinal arch and provides foot inversion. The anterior compartment of the leg contains the dorsiflexors or extensors of the foot. They are the tibialis anterior, extensor digitorum longus, extensor hallucis longus, and peroneus tertius. The lateral compartment contains the peroneals, both longus and brevis. Both groups are innervated by the common peroneal nerve. With its insertion on the medial cuneiform and adjacent base of the first metatarsal, the tibialis anterior surface is a foot inverter, ankle dorsiflexor, and arch supporter. The extensor tendons aid in extension. The peroneus longus lies posterior to the tendon of the peroneus brevis and inserts into the base of the first metatarsal and the medial cuneiform. The peroneus brevis continues more laterally to attach to the base of the fifth metatarsal. The peroneal group is responsible for foot eversion. Thus the integrity of the longitudinal and transverse arches of the foot depend primarily on bony structures and the support derived from the ligaments and aponeurosis and secondarily on the extrinsic musculature originating in the leg during dynamic activity.

Intrinsic Muscles

The only dorsal intrinsic muscle of the foot is the extensor digitorum brevis, which runs from the anterior region of the superior lateral calcaneus to the dorsum of the first four toes. The lateral terminal branch of the deep peroneal nerve innervates the muscle. There are four layers to the plantar intrinsic muscles, all of which are innervated by the medial or lateral plantar nerves. From medial to lateral, the abductor hallucis, flexor digitorum brevis, and abductor digiti minimi constitute the first layer. The muscles arise from the calcaneal tuberosity and insert into the toes. They are important to the dynamic stability of the longitudinal arch.

The quadratus plantae and the lumbricales make up the second layer, and the tendons of the flexor digitorum longus and flexor hallucis longus pass through the region on their way to their respective insertions. The quadratus plantae arises from two heads on the medial and lateral calcaneal tuberosity and terminates in tendinous slips, joining the long flexor tendons to the second, third, fourth, and occasionally fifth toes. The lumbricales arise from the tendon to the flexor digitorum longus and insert into the dorsal aspect of the proximal phalanges. Their function is to flex the metatarsal phalangeal joint and extend the proximal interphalangeal joint. Paralysis or absence of the lumbricales results in hammer toes.

The third layer consists of the adductor hallucis, flexor hallucis brevis, and adductor digiti quinti. Arising from the cuboid and lateral cuneiform, the flexor hallucis brevis divides into medial and lateral components before its insertion into the corresponding aspects of the base of the proximal phalanx of the first toe. The oblique and transverse head of the adductor hallucis insert into the lateral border of the flexor hallucis brevis. The bases of the second, third, and fourth metatarsal head give rise to the oblique head of the adductor hallucis, and the deep transverse metatarsal ligament between the third, fourth, and fifth metatarsal provides site origin for the smaller transverse head. The origin of the flexor digiti minimi is the base of the fifth metatarsal. Together, the tendon of the abductor digit minimi inserts on the lateral side of the base of the proximal phalanx of the fifth toe.

The fourth layer of intrinsic muscles is made up of the plantar and dorsal interossei. Found also in this layer are the tendons of the peroneus longus and tibialis posterior. The four dorsal interossei are bipennate and are located in the intermetatarsal areas. Their function is to abduct the second, third, and fourth toes from the axis through the second metatarsal ray. The three plantar interossei are unipennate and function to adduct the three lateral toes by inserting into the medial sides of the bases of the proximal phalanges of the third, fourth, and fifth toes.

NEUROLOGY

The sciatic nerve provides the motor and sensory innervation of the foot. It divides into the common peroneal and tibial nerves, both of which are derived from the ventral rami, L4–S3, and lie within a common sheath. The smaller component, the common peroneal nerve, divides into superficial and deep components. The superficial peroneal nerve (musculocutaneous) provides cutaneous sensory distribution to the dorsum of the foot, the medial portion of the hallux, the lateral side of the second toe, the medial surface of the third toe, the adjacent sides of the third, fourth, and fifth toes, and the lateral portion of the ankle. The motor portion of the deep peroneal nerve (see Fig. 3) (anterior tibial nerve) supplies the extensor hallucis longus, tibialis anterior, extensor digitorum longus and brevis, peroneus tertius, and sensory innervation of the medial aspect of the second toe and the lateral side of the hallux. The third component of the common peroneal nerve is the sural nerve, which provides sensory distribution to the skin of the lateral malleolus and the fifth toe.

The tibial nerve (posterior tibial or medial popliteal) supplies the heel of the medial sole of the foot, as well as the posterior compartments of the leg. It divides into the medial and lateral plantar nerves (see Fig. 4) and serves the intrinsic muscles of the foot, with the exception of the extensor digitorum brevis. The nerve and its branch provide cutaneous innervation to most of the plantar aspect of the foot. The saphenous, the largest cutaneous branch of the femoral nerve (L2–L4), provides cutaneous innervation to the medial aspect of the foot, often extending as far as the metatarsal phalangeal joint of the hallux. It is the only nerve to the foot that is of nonsciatic origin.

VASCULAR

Arteries

The anterior and posterior arteries, which are the two terminal branches of the popliteal arteries (see Fig. 3), supply the foot. The anterior tibial arteries, in concert with the venae comitantes, pass beneath the superior and inferior extensor retinacula to the dorsum of the foot as the dorsalis pedis artery. The anterior tibial artery also gives rise to the anterior medial and lateral malleolar arteries. The origin of the anastomotic network is formed by the anterior malleolar arteries. The medial and lateral tarsal branches are derived from the dorsalis pedis. The dorsalis pedis gives rise to the arcuate artery and the first dorsal and plantar metatarsal artery.

The larger posterior tibial artery, in accompaniment with the vena comitantes, courses around the medial malleolus, just medial to the medial border of the tendoachilles, and divides into the medial and lateral plantar arteries after passing underneath the flexor retinaculum with its accompanying neurovascular bundle. The smaller medial plantar artery (see Fig. 4) supplies the first and third metatarsal spaces. The larger lateral artery anastomoses with the dorsalis pedis to create the plantar vascular arch, which directs the arterial supply to the lateral four toes, with a smaller contribution to the hallux. The largest branch of the posterior tibial artery is the peroneal artery, which supplies the lateral and posterior aspects of the calcaneus. It anastomoses with the anterior lateral malleolar branches. It is important to bear in mind that there is wide variation between the arterial architectures of the foot and the leg. Up to 15% of individuals may be missing a dorsalis pedis artery, although the posterior tibial is always present.

Veins

The venous drainage system of the foot consists of both superficial and deep branches. The greater and lesser saphenous veins are the principal superficial veins of the lower leg, with a deep plantar venous arch serving as a primary deep drainage system. This arch system empties into the vena comitantes, which ascend to unite in the region of the interosseous membrane and from the popliteal vein, which eventually empties into the femoral vein. It is important to note that both the superficial and deep networks of the veins communicate extensively, particularly near the edge of the ankle and in the distal and medial portion of the leg. The valvular arrangement in the perforating veins enables blood to flow from the superficial veins to the deep network, but not in the opposite direction, under normal conditions. Incompetence of the valves occurs with varicose veins. The long saphenous vein lies just anterior to the medial malleolus and is subject to less anatomic variation than the veins of the upper extremity.

No lymphatic nodes are found within the foot. The dorsal aspect of the foot receives the lymphatic plexus of the digits, with the lymphatic vessels following the course of the saphenous vein to the nodes of the popliteal fossa and then to the inguinal nodes.

BIBLIOGRAPHY

1. Hunter SC, Cappiello WL, Hess GP, Joyce D: Foot problems. In Mellion MB, Walsh WM, Shelton GL: The Team Physician's Handbook. Philadelphia, PA, Hanley & Belfus, 1990, pp 452–463.
2. Riegger CL: Anatomy of the foot and ankle. Phys Ther 68:1802–1814, 1988.
3. Williams PL, Warwick R, Dyson M, Bannister LH (eds): Gray's Anatomy, 37th ed. Edinburgh, Churchill Livingstone, 1989.

Chapter 2

HISTORY AND PHYSICAL EXAMINATION

Richard B. Birrer, M.D., and Michael P. DellaCorte, D.P.M.

The foot and ankle are uniquely adapted to transmit the total body weight to the physical environment. The versatility of these structures, coupled with thick heel and toe pads and the resiliency of the longitudinal transverse arches of the foot, allows concentrated stresses to be dissipated over a large variety of terrain and provide the fine adjustments and balance necessary for walking and other ambulatory activities. The foot and ankle are not immune to the long-term effects of microtrauma from the physical environment or to other general systemic conditions such as arthritis, diabetes, or peripheral vascular disease. Even the shoes that are worn to protect the feet against the ravages of the environment may cause or worsen many foot problems. Thus it becomes imperative, when taking a history and performing a physical examination, not only that feet and ankles be examined but also that the wear of shoes and the stresses on other areas of the body be considered because they may give clues to pathology affecting feet.

A thorough and successful evaluation of the foot is contingent upon solid knowledge of anatomy, physiology, and biomechanics. The history should be taken in four parts: chief complaint, history of the present illness, past medical history, and review of systems.

HISTORY

Chief Complaint/History of the Present Illness

The chief complaint should be described by the patient. The history of the present illness should include the time and type of onset,

intensity, duration, quality, conditions that relieve or aggravate the symptom(s), and whether the problem is referred to other regions of the foot or lower extremity. As examples, consider the acute, severe, localized pain of gout, the intermittent claudication of peripheral vascular disease associated with walking, the relief of osteoid osteoma pain by aspirin, the burning pain of metatarsalgia with hyperkeratosis, and the pain of initial weight bearing in the early morning related to plantar heel-spur syndrome. It is often helpful to categorize complaints as primary or secondary and to go through detailed questioning about each. If there is a question of trauma, then the mechanism and the injury must be fully elucidated. Was there a direct blow to the dorsum of the foot? Did the foot begin to hurt after a long run on a rough surface (e.g., stone bruise)? It is particularly important to determine whether there is forced inversion or eversion of the foot with or without associated plantar flexion or dorsiflexion. The time at which the injury occurred, whether there was any immediate therapy, and what the outcome was are also very important. If the injury is a chronic one, has there been any rehabilitation, prolonged immobilization, or recurrent instability or symptomatology since the time of the injury? Previous treatment modalities should be investigated. These include medications, orthotics, laboratory and radiographic evaluations, and, in the event of surgery, the outcome.

Past Medical History

It is important to get a thorough past medical history, including family background.

This history should detail allergies, with care being taken to include specific items used in the treatment of the lower extremity, such as iodine (Betadine preparations), local anesthetics, and tape. Medication history, including use of tobacco and alcohol, previous hospitalizations, and any recent fevers, is an essential component of the complete history. The family background should be checked for vascular disease, arthritis, gout, hypertension, cancer, cardiovascular disease, and bleeding problems.

Review of Systems

Since feet can present the first clinical evidence of systemic pathology, the patient should be asked about thyroid disease, peripheral vascular disease, vasculitis, gout, psoriasis, diabetes, malignancy, collagen vascular disease, and arthritis of any etiology. A number of neurologic problems affecting the back could present themselves only with foot findings; herniated nucleus pulposus, spina bifida, spinal cord tumors, neurofibromatosis, and Friedreich's ataxia commonly involve the foot and do so before other symptoms become evident. The review of systems should also highlight history of congenital or childhood infectious problems (e.g., Charcot-Marie-Tooth disease, poliomyelitis, clubfoot) and the presence of edema (e.g., hepatic, renal, or cardiac disease). Finally, during the general systemic review, an attempt should be made to determine the patient's psychological perception of the foot problem. For instance, what is the individual's pain threshold? Is there an element of secondary gain, malingery, or hypochondriasis present?

Personal History

An occupational and hobby history should include the amount of weight bearing that the patient undergoes during the work day (e.g., delivery jobs, sanitation, mechanics), whether the patient has a sitting or desk job, and what type of shoe gear is worn to work versus what type of shoe gear is worn at work. Lastly, if the patient is an athlete, a full athletic history should be taken in terms of the type and amount of sports activity in which the patient participates on a regular basis. Any regimen changes (e.g., increased or decreased distances, change in surface or footwear) are critical. Past injuries and their treatments should be fully reviewed, as should the gear that the patient wears, the athletic surfaces that the patient plays on, and the amount of time per week that the patient spends on the athletic endeavor.

THE PHYSICAL EXAMINATION

Observation/Vital Signs

The physical exam begins when the patient walks through the physician's door. The patient should be asked to ambulate to and fro, turn 180 degrees, and repeat the movement. The same activities should then be performed on the heels and balls of the feet. During weight-bearing activity, any deformities should be noted such as differences in the width or length of both feet, heel varus or valgus, calf atrophy, splayfoot, varicose veins, and intoeing or out-toeing, which may suggest internal tibial torsion or anteversion of the femoral necks in children. Observation that takes note of posture, gait, antalgia, shuffling, steppage, or other deformity is important. The patient's clothing, from the waist down, should be removed and the exam repeated. Note carefully the position and function of the feet and ankles as the patient undresses. Weight bearing is a useful stress test for underlying pathology. The patient's vital signs are recorded. The exam should then begin with the patient seated on the exam table with shoes and socks off.

General Inspection

In the normally relaxed position there are mild plantar flexion and inversion of the feet. Dorsiflexion and eversion are characteristic of a spastic flatfoot. The medial longitudinal arch produces a perceptible dome on the dorsum of the foot, which extends from the calcaneus to the first metatarsal head. At rest, while not weight bearing, this arch is more prominent. However, when it is excessively high, it is termed pes cavus; when absent, pes planus. A collapsed arch is suggestive of neuropathic injury or a Charcot joint. In children, there may be some medial inclination of the forefoot on the hindfoot, termed forefoot adductus, or the hindfoot may be in excessive valgus or varus position. The number of toes should be noted. They should appear straight, flat, and proportional to one another when compared with those of the other foot. Overlapping toes should be noted because they can be suggestive of an underlying hammer toe and/or bunion.

Vascular Examination

Evaluation of the vascular network includes the dorsalis pedis, posterior tibialis, and popliteal and femoral pulses. They are graded 0 to 4, with 3 to 4 being normal. The femoral pulse lies just inferior to the inguinal ligament at a point midway between the anterior superior iliac spine and the pubic tubercle. The superficial dorsalis pedis pulse is easily palpated on the dorsum of the foot between the extensor digitorum longus and hallucis longus tendon. The posterior tibial artery is palpated just posterior to the medial malleoli between the tibialis posterior tendon and the flexor digitorum longus tendon. The popliteal pulse can be found by pressing the fingers of both hands up into the popliteal fossa medial to the lateral biceps femoris tendon while the knee is actively extended.

The capillary refill time (normally 3–5 seconds) should be determined by compression of the toe tufts until they blanch. Prolongation of the time it takes for normal pink coloration to return following release is synonymous with vascular disease. Elevation and dependency tests can also be used to assess pedal circulation. Normally there is no pallor (grade 0) after elevating the foot to 60 degrees for 1 minute. Definite pallor in 60 seconds is grade 1, pallor in 30–60 seconds is grade II, pallor in less than 30 seconds is grade III, and pallor without elevation is grade IV. Immediately after the elevation test, the patient should sit up and hang the feet over the examining table edge. Severe ischemia is denoted by color return requiring more than 40 seconds of dependency, moderated occlusive disease if 15–25 seconds are necessary, and normal circulation if color returns in 10–15 seconds. If either test is abnormal, further vascular evaluation should include Doppler and thermography studies. The retrograde filling (Trendelenburg) test is used to assess valvular competency in the communicating veins as well as in the saphenous systems. The great saphenous vein is occluded by a tourniquet on the upper thigh for 20–25 seconds after the leg has been drained of venous blood through elevation. During standing there should be slow filling of the saphenous vein from below as the femoral artery pushes blood through the capillary bed into the venous system. Rapid filling of the superficial veins indicates incompetent communicating venous valves. The tourniquet is then released. Sudden additional filling of the superficial system suggests incompetent valves of the saphenous vein.

Neurologic Examination

The neurologic exam can be cursory unless there is any underlying pathology, such as low back pain or diabetes. The exam should include reflexes of both the Achilles (ankle jerk S1–S2), and prepatellar (knee jerk L2–L4) tendons. It is important to assess vibratory sensations, since they are usually the first to be diminished in diabetic neuropathy. With the patient's eyes closed, a tuning fork is successfully placed on each digit. The sensation should be the same bilaterally. Soft touch and pain should also be evaluated. Check the patient's reliability with a nonvibrating tuning fork or the hub of the needle. The L4 dermatome extends from the medial aspect of the leg to the medial malleolus and the medial side of the foot (Fig. 1). The L5 dermatome covers the lateral side of the leg and the dorsum of the foot (Fig. 2). The S1 dermatome covers the lateral portion of the foot (Fig. 3). If any gait abnormality is noted upon the patient's arrival in the office, then further function tests should be performed, such as heel-toe gait, balance function, and heel-to-shin testing. Sensory

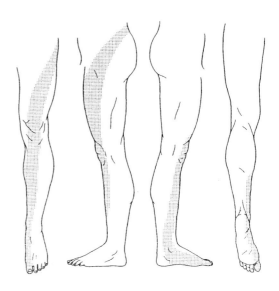

FIGURE 1. L4 dermatome. (From Wienir MA: Limb radicular pain and sensory disturbance. Spine: State of the Art Reviews 2:533–564, 1988, with permission.)

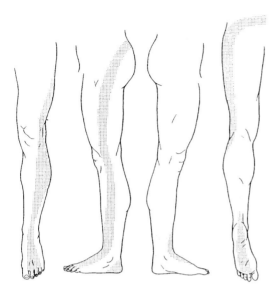

FIGURE 2.   L5 dermatome. (From Wienir MA: Limb radicular pain and sensory disturbance. Spine: State of the Art Reviews 2:533–564, 1988, with permission.)

testing consists of each peripheral nerve that innervates the dorsum of the foot (saphenous on the medial side, peroneal on the dorsum side, and sural on the lateral side) and the L4–L5–S1 dermatomes. The L4 dermatome

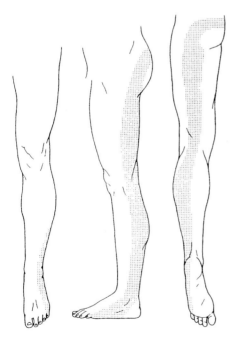

FIGURE 3.   S1 dermatome. (From Wienir MA: Limb radicular pain and sensory disturbance. Spine: State of the Art Reviews 2:533–564, 1988, with permission.)

extends from the medial aspect of the leg to the medial malleolus on the medial side of the foot. The L5 dermatome covers the lateral side of the leg and the dorsum of the foot. Motor testing can also be accomplished, but it is easier to do during the musculoskeletal part of the physical examination.

Dermatologic Examination

The web spaces should be inspected for any sign of inflammation or vesicles indicative of a tinea infection. Next, the skin of the dorsum of the foot should be visually inspected. It should be smooth and nonthickened and should contain hair follicles, particularly over the toes. A loss of hair on the toes is indicative of poor arterial supply to the digits (e.g., peripheral vascular disease, diabetes). The plantar surface, especially the ball and the bed, contain thickened areas in order to accommodate weight bearing. Abnormal lichenification and thickening of the skin over the metatarsal heads or the medial border of the hallux occur in response to the bearing of abnormal amounts of weight (e.g., tyloma or heloma). The location of such lesions should be carefully noted. Skin color is typically dark pink during weight bearing, becoming lighter during non-weight-bearing activity. If, during dependence, the foot becomes deep red, indicating dependent rubor, small-vessel disease is suggested. Cyanosis, skin atrophy, and ulceration are suggestive of vascular disease. Medial ulcerations are more common in venous disease, whereas lateral ulcerations are more typical of arterial disease. Both occur principally at the level of the malleoli. Inspection should be concluded by noting whether there is localized or generalized edema of the foot or ankle. Unilateral localized edema is highly suggestive of trauma or infection (e.g., tinea) if there are also associated erythema and warmth. Bilateral swelling is more suggestive of hepatic, cardiac, or renal pathology or pelvic obstruction to venous return. Occasionally, unilateral edema can follow congenital absence of lymph glands (Milroy's disease) or obstruction due to primary or secondary carcinoma. The toenails should be carefully inspected for dystrophia, erythema, discoloration, pitting, and deformity. Excessive growth of a nail along with its medial or lateral margins (unguis incarnatus) can produce erythema, edema, and secondary infection. Clubbing of the nails suggests cardiopulmonary compromise.

Biomechanical Examination

Biomechanics is the application of mechanical laws to living structures, specifically to the locomotor system of the human body. The biomechanical exam is probably the most difficult part of the lower-extremity assessment and must include not only the foot and ankle but also the knee and hip. The anatomic position for lower-extremity biomechanical examination places the patient standing, erect, with feet perpendicular to the body and at the normal angle and base of gait. It is best to start with the patient lying supine on the examination table. Palpate the anterior superior iliac spines, and measure the distance between them and the ipsilateral medial malleolus in order to determine limb length. A true limb-length discrepancy of 5 mm or more can cause significant functional and structural problems. Measuring from a nonfixed point (e.g., umbilicus) will detect any apparent limb-length discrepancy due to pelvic tilt.

It is not necessary to measure joint motion per se, but it is necessary to know if a particular motion is in the abnormal range. Therefore, both sides should be tested for comparison. One should note the internal and external rotation of the hip during extension and flexion. This transverse plane motion should be equal in both the extended and flexed positions, and both hips should have the same range of motion.

The position of the knee should be noted (i.e., varus, valgus, recurvatum); mild valgus is normal.

There are three body planes in which the foot and ankle function: transverse, sagittal, and frontal. Motion can occur in one plane, two planes, or all three planes. Dorsiflexion is a pure sagittal plane motion. It is described as the top of the foot moving closer to the anterior leg. Plantarflexion, the opposing sagittal plane motion, occurs when the foot moves away from the anterior leg. The two frontal plane motions are inversion and eversion. Inversion occurs when the bottom of the foot turns toward the midline of the body. Eversion is the opposite action, i.e., the bottom of the foot turns away from the midline of the body. Abduction and adduction are the two pure transverse plane motions. Abduction occurs when the foot rotates away from the midline of the body. Adduction is described as the foot moving toward the midline of the body.

Ankle joint range of motion should be evaluated. The hinge joint of the ankle provides 20 degrees of dorsiflexion and 50 degrees of plantar flexion. In order to assess this motion, it is essential to stabilize the subtalar joint by fixating the calcaneus and inverting the forefoot so that it locks into the hindfoot, thus prohibiting forefoot motion. The patient should be sitting at the edge of the examination table with the knees bent, relaxing the gastrocnemius and the soleus muscles. The forefoot should then be gripped and the foot both plantarflexed and dorsiflexed. The relationship of the lateral aspect of the foot and the posterior aspect of the leg are the reference points to determine ankle joint range of motion (Fig. 4). A small amount of lateral talar tilt between the malleoli can occur in full plantar flexion under normal conditions. This is because the narrow posterior portion of the talus does not fit tightly into the mortise formed by the tibia and fibula. However, in dorsiflexion the talus is held snugly between the two malleoli. Edema of an extra-articular or intra-articular location will reduce or constrict normal ankle motions. End points will feel boggy. Less than 10 degrees of dorsiflexion suggests an equinus condition. If a patient exhibits less than 10 degrees of dorsiflexion, it is important to note if the equinus is soft

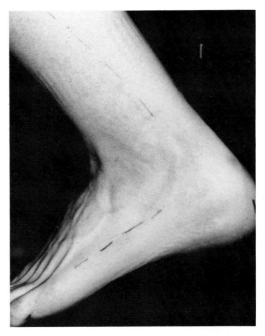

FIGURE 4. Testing for equinus: 1. Bisect the lateral leg. 2. Bisect the lateral foot. 3. Place subtalar joint in neutral position. 4. Patient actively dorsiflexes foot. 5. Ten degrees of dorsiflexion rules out equinus.

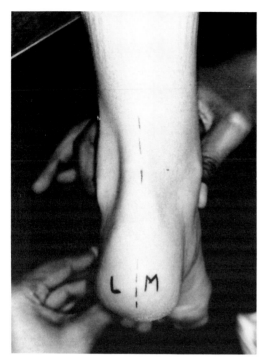

FIGURE 5. Neutral position of subtalar joint. The line bisecting the posterior leg and the line bisecting the posterior calcaneus should be in line.

Pain and restriction of motion are suggestive of either possible fracture acutely or degenerative joint disease or arthritis more chronically. Subtalar mobility is enhanced in the younger patient.

Triplanar motion is motion that deviates from all three body planes. Two major joints of the foot—the subtalar and midtarsal—are triplanar joints. The triplanar motions are termed pronation and supination. The pronatory supinatory axis begins posterior, plantar, and lateral, and it ends medial anterior and dorsal. Around this axis occur the motions of pronation (Fig. 6) (consisting of abduction, dorsiflexion, and eversion) and supination (Fig. 7) (consisting of adduction, plantarflexion, and inversion). The subtalar joint has one axis around which triplanar motion exists. Three times more motion occurs in the transverse and frontal planes than the sagittal plane due to the greater axis deviation from the transverse and frontal planes. The midtarsal joint (MTJ) consists of the talonavicular and calcaneocuboid joints and contains two axes: longitudinal (LMTJ) and oblique (OMTJ).

tissue or is osseous in nature; this is done by reducing the stretch of gastrocnemius through knee flexion. No change in dorsiflexion suggests an osseous lesion (see Chapter 12).

For this part of the examination the patient should be rolled to a prone position on the examination table with the feet hanging over the edge. The table should be elevated to a comfortable height for the examiner's manipulation of the person's foot. The patient's subtalar joint should be moved into neutral position. Essential to understanding normal lower-extremity function is subtalar joint (STJ) neutral position. Neutral position is defined as the position in which the joint functions best (Fig. 5). To determine the STJ neutral position, put the joint through its total excursion of motion while palpating the head of the talus anteriorly within the ankle mortise and moving the calcaneus in a pronatory and supinatory direction. When you feel the change of direction of that motion, the joint is in its neutral position. Generally, the STJ has twice as much supination as pronation—20 degrees and 10 degrees, respectively. Subtalar motion derived from the concerted activities of the foot allows functioning on uneven surfaces.

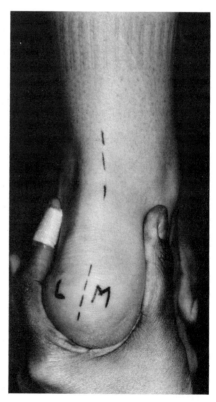

FIGURE 6. Subtalar joint pronation. L = lateral; M = medial.

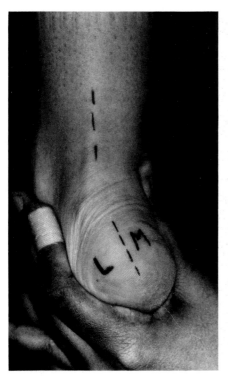

FIGURE 7.   Subtalar joint supination.

Both axes are triplanar. The LMTJ has more motion in all three planes. Deviation from the triplanar motion, at either the STJ, the OMTJ, or the LMTJ, can occur due to rearfoot or forefoot deformities intrinsically created at birth or by compensation of foot abnormalities in the proximal lower extremity.

Once the foot is in neutral position, the amount of calcaneal varus/valgus should be evaluated off weight bearing. It is highly unusual for the calcaneus to be in a valgus position, but it does occur. Next, the forefoot-to-rearfoot configuration should be noted for the amount of varus or valgus at the midtarsal joint. This is done by sighting from the rear of the calcaneus down the forefoot along the plane formed by the metatarsals (Fig. 8). The midtarsal joint does not have a neutral position; it is most stable when maximally pronated. This can be achieved by "loading" the lateral column of the foot, which is performed by placing your thumb below the fifth metatarsal head and applying force to stimulate weight bearing. Ideally, the patient's foot should exhibit a small amount of rearfoot varus in the calcaneus, maybe 3 degrees, and a parallel midtarsal joint or forefoot-to-rearfoot position, so that there appears to be no deviation in the inverted

or everted position when one sights down the calcaneus. Once a deformity is identified, it must be determined whether the deformity is fixed or flexible. Fixed deformities of the foot can be uniplanar, triplanar, or a combination of both. The sagittal-plane fixed deformities are pes calcaneus (calcaneus in dorsiflexed position) and equinus (rearfoot is plantarflexed). Frontal-plane deformities are varus (fixed inversion) and valgus (fixed eversion), which can occur at the forefoot, rearfoot, tibia, or knee. Transverse fixed deformities include abductus (foot pointing away from the body) and adductus (pointing toward the body). Triplane deformities include supinatus and pronatus.

The first metatarsophalangeal joint can be flexed 45 degrees and extended 70–90 degrees. The proximal interphalangeal joint of the first toe is capable of 70–90 degrees of flexion. Reduced motion in the first toe (i.e., hallux limitus or rigidus) is usually reflected in an abnormal gait consisting of a shortened "toe-off/push-off" phase, which is usually protective and antalgic. In the four lateral toes, only the metatarsophalangeal joint can actively extend, whereas the distal and proximal interphalangeal joints are capable of active flexion. Thus, in assessment of the range of motion of the lesser toes, passive extension and flexion of the proximal and distal interphalangeal as well as of the metatarsophalangeal joints are essential. Very often, subtle deformities such as claw toe or hammer toe can be elicited.

The patient should now stand in front of the practitioner and be barefoot in a comfortable position for determination of the angle and base of gait. Angle of gait is defined as the angle of the foot to the line of progression (Fig. 9). The line of progression is a straight

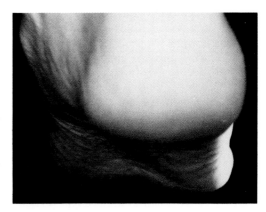

FIGURE 8.   Forefoot varus. (Note the inversion of the forefoot in relation to the rearfoot.)

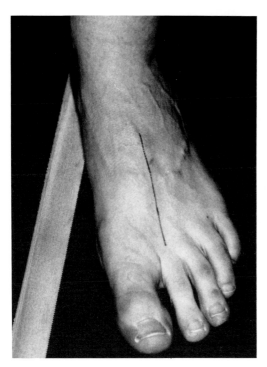

FIGURE 9. Angle of gait. White tape represents the line of progression; the line on the foot is the center reference point of the foot. Normal angle of gait is 10–15° abducted.

line in the direction that the patient is walking. The normal angle of gait is 5–10 degrees abducted. Note if the patient is in-toed or out-toed. Base of gait is the distance between the right and left malleoli as one foot swings past the other during gait. Normal base of gait is 1–2 cm during swing phase. Have the patient stand with his or her back to you and evaluate the position of the calcaneus. Neutral calcaneal stance position and resting calcaneal stance position should then be determined. Is there significant valgus in stance? Custom-made foot orthotics can be prescribed to reduce or correct abnormalities discovered in the biomechanical exam. The biomechanical goal in treatment of the patient is to decrease the amount of foot and leg compensation secondary to poorly aligned joints or structural deformities.

Another method of assessing foot biomechanics is the use of the Harris foot mat. The mat is an inked rubber sheet with elevated squares of rubber at various heights so that areas of increasing pressure bring more and more inked rubber edges to the paper. Thus a printout of the loading pattern can be made. Frequently, excessive loading under the metatarsal heads becomes more noticeable with

this test. If this mat is unavailable, Betadine solution can be applied to the plantar aspect of the foot, and the patient can then stand on a piece of white paper, providing a two-dimensional impression of the foot. A plaster of Paris cast of the foot will give a true three-dimensional impression, which is necessary for the fabrication of functional foot orthotics.

The Gait Cycle

The ideal conditions for normal gait require a level pelvis, legs of equal length, knee joint axis in the frontal plane (i.e., knees facing straight ahead), knees and ankles directly over each other, and legs straight and perpendicular to the foot, with the first and fifth rays in the same plane (i.e., level) and rays 2, 3, and 4 and finally the ankle joint having a minimum of 10 degrees of dorsiflexion available when the STJ is in neutral position and the MTJ is maximally pronated. Any abnormalities in the above lead to changes in foot function and gait.

The gait cycle describes normal walking (Fig. 10). (Running creates a variation in the cycle.) The gait cycle observed during walking consists of two parts: a swing phase and a stance phase. The swing phase is the time when the foot does not touch the ground and is swinging forward. This constitutes approximately one third of the cycle. The stance phase is the time when the foot makes contact with the ground. This constitutes approximately two thirds of the gait cycle.

The stance phase can be divided into three phases, beginning with heel contact and ending with toe-off of the same foot. The first division of the stance phase is the contact phase, which begins when heel contact is completed with full forefoot loading. It constitutes the first 27% of the stance phase. At heel strike, the foot is inverted to the ground, the leg internally rotates, and the STJ pronates, allowing the foot to become a "mobile adapter" to uneven ground. STJ pronation also allows the knee to flex, enhancing shock absorption (Fig. 10a).

The second division of the stance phase is midstance, which occurs when the forefoot and rearfoot are in contact with the ground. It begins with full forefoot loading and ends with heel-off. Midstance constitutes 40% of the stance phase. During midstance, the STJ begins resupination so that the forefoot becomes a rigid lever for propulsion. At the midpoint of midstance, the subtalar joint is in the neutral position, and the opposite leg is swinging by (Fig. 10b).

The last division of the stance phase is the propulsion phase, which begins with heel-off and ends with toe-off. Propulsion constitutes 33% of the stance phase. Weight is transferred during the contact and midstance phases from the lateral heel to medial forefoot so that during propulsion, stress is passed out through the first and second toes as a rigid level for propulsion. Stress then passes to the opposite foot at heel contact, and the cycle starts over again (Fig. 10c).

To enhance smooth walking, six elements are needed. (1) Pelvic rotation—the hip of the swinging limb rotates around the stance-phase limb, allowing for less drop of the center of gravity and thus decreasing shock at heel contact. (2) Pelvic drop occurs during midstance, and the swing-phase limb is lowered approximately 5 degrees when swinging by the stance-phase limb; hence the center of gravity need not be raised as high for a smoother walk. (3) Knee flexion occurs at contact to reduce the shock of heel contact and to decrease the amount necessary to raise the center of gravity. (4) The ankle joint plantarflexes, reducing the amount of shock the foot encounters at heel strike. (5) The subtalar joint and midtarsal joint go through their range of motion for smooth walking throughout the gait cycle. (6) The body displaces its weight laterally so that the torso is over the weight-bearing foot. The distal end of the femur is angled inward for less lateral displacement of the body, which leads to a smoother walk. In addition, the upper body rotates 180 degrees opposite that of the lower extremity so as to reduce the transverse and sagittal motions of the lower extremity.

Deviation from the above-described normal gait cycle components results in abnormalities in foot function, which progress to foot deformities (e.g., bunions, hammer toes, flatfoot) (see Chapter 12).

Musculoskeletal Examination

Palpation of the foot is easily begun with the first toe. The metatarsal and metatarsophalangeal joints are readily palpated. Carefully palpate the soft tissue overlying the joint,

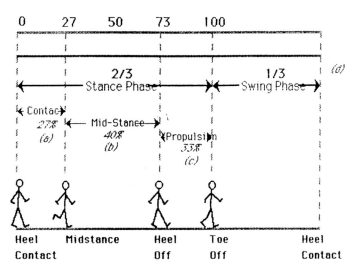

FIGURE 10. Gait cycle—walking.

noting its angulation and the presence or absence of underlying bursal inflammation, which may be due to pressure, friction, or urate deposition. More proximally along the medial border of the foot is the prominent navicular tubercle. A localized trigger point or tenderness is often associated with antalgia in children and is suggestive of osteochondritis dissecans of the navicular (Kohler's). Flexion and inversion of the foot cause the tibialis posterior to stand out (L5 ramus). Directly posterior to the tibialis posterior tendon, the flexor digitorum longus tendon is best palpated by resisting plantar flexion of the patient's toes while the calcaneus is stabilized. The tendon of the flexor hallucis longus cannot be palpated but can be tested by opposition of plantar flexion of the great toe. Medially, the large, strong, and wide deltoid ligament is usually not palpable in the space inferior to the medial malleolus. Most proximally, the prominent medial malleolus articulates with one third of the medial side of the talus.

On the lateral aspect of the foot, both the metatarsal phalangeal joint and the head of the fifth metatarsal bone are easily palpated. Overlying the head of the fifth metatarsal bone is a bursa, which, due to its superficial nature, can easily become inflamed, a condition commonly referred to as "tailor's bunion." As one travels proximally along the shaft of the fifth metatarsal, its flared base, the styloid process, becomes evident. The tendon of the peroneus brevis inserts into the styloid process. Between the styloid process and the cuboid bone is a depression that contains the peroneus longus tendon as it travels to the medial plantar surface of the foot. As one continues to move more proximally to the calcaneus, its peroneal tubercle, which separates the peroneus longus and brevis tendons, is easily noted. The tubercle is just distal to the lateral malleolus and is usually about 5 cm in length, though it varies from patient to patient. The peronei can be assessed by opposing plantar flexion and eversion, with pressure against the head and shaft of the fifth metatarsal.

The distal portion of the fibula constitutes the lateral malleolus. It extends more distally than the medial malleolus and is more effective in preventing eversion injury. The dome of the talus can be appreciated by plantar flexing the foot, with the examiner's thumb placed on the anterior lateral portion of the malleolus. By application of a small amount of inversion force, more of the talar dome can be appreciated. The sinus tarsi area can be felt by placing the thumb just anterior to the lateral malleolus and the soft tissue depression, which is filled by a superficial fat pad and the deeper extensor digitorum brevis muscle. With rare exception, as in the case of ankle trauma with diastasis, the inferior portion of the tibiofibular joint can be appreciated. It lies immediately proximal to the talus and is fortified by very strong anterior inferior tibiofibular ligaments. The anterior talofibular ligament transverses the sinus tarsi and is the first ligament torn in inversion ankle sprains. Pathology of the subtalar complex, such as fracture or rheumatoid arthritis, produces deep tenderness on palpation of the sinus tarsi. The extensor digitorum brevis can be appreciated by having the patient voluntarily extend the toes while the sinus tarsi is palpated.

The lateral collateral ligaments (anterior talofibular, calcaneal, fibular, and posterior talofibular) are not distinctly palpable under normal conditions. Their functional integrity can best be assessed through a number of ankle joint stress tests. In order to test the integrity of the anterior talofibular ligament, plantar flexion and inversion should be performed. The production of pain in the region of the sinus tarsi is highly suggestive of a sprain of the ligament. Greater degrees of pain that are more diffuse suggest that the calcaneofibular ligament may also be involved. Tibiotalar stability can be assessed by performing the anterior drawer test (Fig. 11). With one hand on the anterior aspect of the tibia and with the calcaneus in the palm of the other hand, the calcaneus and talus are drawn anteriorly, while the distal tibia is pushed posteriorly. There is no pain and only imperceptible movement under normal conditions. Anterior displacement of the talus and calcaneus by more than 3–5 mm or a difference of greater than 0.5 mm between ankles is highly suggestive of a rupture of the anterior talofibular ligament. A soft end-point or the perception of a "clunk" may be appreciated and is also considered to be a positive

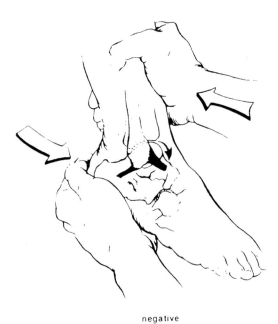

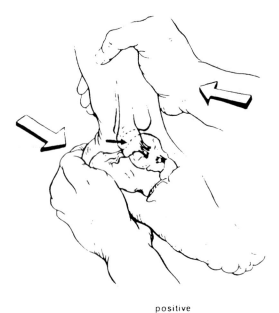

negative   positive

FIGURE 11.   The drawer test.

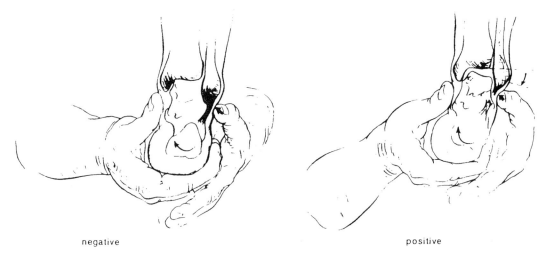

negative   positive

FIGURE 12. The talar tilt stress test.

sign. Reversing the procedure assesses the stability in the posterior plane. It is important both that the anteroposterior muscles surrounding the ankle are completely relaxed and that the ankle is positioned 90 degrees to the leg, because it is often impossible to demonstrate even a significantly positive anterior drawer sign in the plantar flexed position. The results should always be compared to the normal side. If the injury is acute, the infiltration of 5–10 cc of 1% lidocaine in the joint opposite to the side of injury with additional infiltration of the involved ligament(s) is often useful.

The talar tilt or inversion/eversion stress test can be used to assess integrity of the lateral as well as the medial ligaments of the ankle (Fig. 12). The normal angle of talar tilt is between 3 and 23 degrees, and a 5–10 degree difference between the ankles is considered within normal limits. In the case of a questionable lateral tear, an inversion force is applied to the talus with the foot in equinus. Opening up of the ankle mortise in this manner is suggestive of a tear of two or more of the lateral compartments. Repeat of the stress test with the foot in the neutral position and production of a tilt suggest concomitant rupture of the calcaneofibular ligament. It is usually not necessary to perform a drawer test if integrity of the deltoid ligament is questionable. In this case, an eversion force is applied and an abnormal gap of the ankle mortise denotes ligament rupture. Each of these clinical tests can be confirmed by simultaneous stress radiographs.

The hindfoot can best be examined by placing the heel in the palm of the hand and by the thumb and the index finger in the contralateral soft tissue depressions on either side of the tendoachillis. The posterior third of the calcaneus is easily appreciated. As one moves plantar, the bone normally flares at its outer base. On the medial plantar aspect of the calcaneus, there is a medial tubercle, which tends to be broad and large and which provides attachment for the flexor digitorum brevis, plantar aponeurosis, and abductor hallucis muscle. A tender medial tubercle may suggest a heel spur. More posterior tenderness along the calcaneus, especially in children, is suggestive of epiphysitis (Sever's disease). The large Achilles tendon, which represents the combined tendon of the gastrocnemius and soleus muscles, inserts into the posterior calcaneus. Its integrity can be assessed by direct palpation, by having the patient either jump up and down on the balls of the feet or walk on the toes, and by the Thompson-Doherty squeeze test (Fig. 13). Squeezing the calf, which normally produces plantar flexion, produces markedly decreased motion or none at all. If the tendon has been acutely ruptured, there is often a palpable gap, which is painful and tender where the rupture has occurred. Between the overlying skin and the insertion of the tendoachillis lies the calcaneal bursa, which can become inflamed following excessive direct pressure or secondary damage to the tendoachillis. High heels and tight shoes are frequently responsible. Between the tendoachillis and the posterior superior aspect of the calcaneus lies the retrocalcaneal bursa. As with the calcaneal bursa, it can become inflamed following tendinitis or severe contusion of the calcaneus.

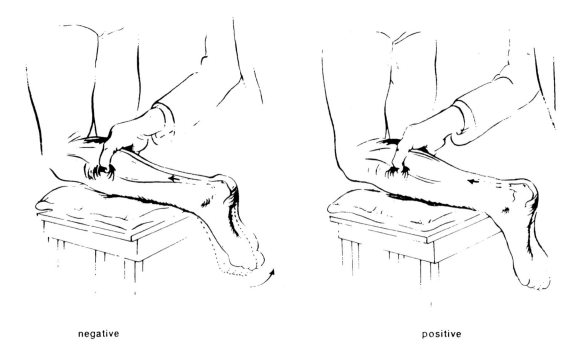

negative   positive

FIGURE 13.   The Thompson-Doherty squeeze test for integrity of the Achilles tendon.

Examination of the plantar surface of the foot is somewhat difficult due to the thickness of the overlying skin, as well as the supportive connective tissue layers of the arches and fat pad. With the lower extremity in extension and the calf of the leg supported by one of the examiner's hands, the sole of the foot is gently palpated. Firm pressure at the first metatarsal head reveals two small sesamoid bones lying within the tendon of the flexor hallucis brevis. Tenderness suggests sesamoiditis, which can be aggravated during the toe-off portion of normal gait. During palpation, one should assess the presence or absence of tenderness and the size and location of each head.

Proximal to the metatarsal heads lies the plantar fascia, or aponeurosis. It should feel smooth and nontender. Tender trigger points may indicate plantar fasciitis, whereas palpation of discrete nodules suggests a Dupuytren's type contracture (plantar fibromatosis) in the foot. Such nodules should be distinguished from more superficial ones, typical of corns and warts. Each of the metatarsal interspaces should be carefully palpated for tenderness and swelling. Identification of a tender trigger between metatarsals is suggestive of neuroma, termed Morton's neuroma if in the third interspace.

The most visible portion of the foot is the dorsum or extensor surface. During weight bearing, the toes should be straight and flat. Metatarsal phalangeal joint hyperextension with flexion of the proximal and distal interphalangeal joints is termed claw toe, which typically involves all toes and is usually associated with pes cavus deformity. Constant frictional irritation by the shoes on the flexed interphalangeal joints produces dorsal callosities over the involved toes. On the plantar surface, callosities often affect the metatarsal heads and the tips of the toes, particularly the second, due to excessive amounts of weight bearing and a more plantar position of one or more bones. Hyperextension of both the metatarsal phalangeal and distal interphalangeal joints is associated with proximal interphalangeal joint flexion and is termed swan neck deformity. Flexion of the proximal interphalangeal joint produces a hammer toe deformity. This malformation usually involves the second toe and is denoted by a proximal interphalangeal joint callosity due to shoe friction.

The shafts of the metatarsal should be palpated for localized trigger points and swelling. There are a number of soft tissue structures, which should also be noted. Resisted dorsiflexion and inversion of the foot make palpation of the tibialis anterior tendon easy as it courses between the malleoli most medially. With opposed extension of the big toe at the distal phalanx, the extensor hallucis longus tendon becomes evident. It is lateral to the tibialis anterior tendon. If the pressure is applied before the interphalangeal joint, the extensor hallucis brevis is also tested. Resisted extension of the toes facilitates palpation of the extensor digitorum longus tendon, which lies lateral to the extensor hallucis longus. It is most easily felt where it crosses the ankle joint before it divides into its four tendinous insertions at the dorsal bases of the distal phalanges of the four lesser toes. Muscle formation should be grossly tested by having the patient invert and evert, abduct and adduct, and dorsiflex and plantarflex against the resistance of the examiner's hands. Toes should also be flexed and extended against resistance. Muscle strength is usually graded on a 0 (no movement) to 5 (normal) scale.

Athletic Considerations

Athletic evaluation should include treadmill evaluation, ideally with video, or watching the patient walk and/or run. Running movements such as cutting and figure of eights should be evaluated. If the athlete is a cyclist, a stationary trainer should be used. This equipment allows the examiner to see, dynamically, what is actually occurring during this activity. With the treadmill, the patient can be evaluated in shorts from the posterior. The patient should be barefoot, in athletic shoe gear, without devices, and with devices if appropriate. In addition to watching the patient participate in his or her athletic endeavor, it is also important to examine the athlete's foot gear.

Evaluation of Footwear

Shoe gear evaluation is essential in the investigation of a foot problem. The investigation should include not only the presumed culprit but also a cross sampling of all footwear regularly used by the patient. Does the footwear accurately fit the feet? Are the shoes loose, tight, shallow, or deep? The shoe is carefully inspected for defects (Fig. 14). Excessive in-toeing causes pronounced amounts of wear on the lateral border of the sole and heel of the shoes. Hallux rigidus often causes a markedly oblique crease of the forepart of the shoe due to toe-off on the lateral side of the foot. The prominence of the talar head in individuals with flat feet tends to produce broken medial counters, whereas individuals with footdrop tend to scuff the shoes during the swing phase in ambulation. Not just the outside of the shoe but the inside as well should be carefully examined for protruding seams, nails, rivets, or wrinkled shoe lining. Very often a visible external convexity will have a concomitant internal concavity corresponding to the hallux or the distal interphalangeal joints of the toes. The examiner should look for wear areas posteriorly, medially, and laterally. Such deformities are often associated with callus or corn formation. Look at the shoe from the rear, and inspect the cant to the heel cup area. Does the shoe fit perpendicular to the sole, or is it inverted or everted? This gives evidence as to the type of abnormal biomechanics: if the shoe is severely everted, pronation is compensatory; if the shoe is very inverted, a rearfoot varus position exists. Next, look at the sole of the shoes and the wear pattern. If the patient

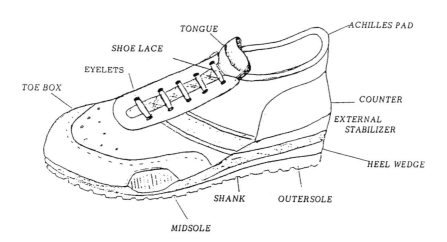

FIGURE 14. Anatomy of a shoe.

is not propulsing off, there will be no wear in the toe area. The type of material from which the shoe is constructed should be noted. Leather is more resilient and flexible than synthetic materials, which, in addition, tend to be allergenic. The height of the heal and the dimensions of the last should be recorded.

SUMMARY

Following the history and physical evaluation, a detailed problem list should be created based on the findings. An assessment and a treatment plan are then formulated for each problem.

BIBLIOGRAPHY

1. Bates B: A Guide to Physical Examination, 3rd ed. Philadelphia, J.B. Lippincott, 1983, pp 345–347, pp 498–503.
2. Czerniecki JM: Foot and ankle biomechanics in walking and running: A review. Am J Phys Med Rehabil 67:246–252, 1988.
3. Hoppenfeld S: Physical Examination of the Spine and Extremities. New York, Appleton-Century-Crofts, Inc., 1976, pp 197–236.
4. Nuber GW: Biomechanics of the foot and ankle during gait. Clin Sports Med 7:1–14, 1988.
5. Oatis CA: Biomechanics of the foot and ankle under static conditions. Phys Ther 68:1815–1821, 1988.
6. Wienir MA (ed): Spinal Segmental Pain and Sensory Disturbance. Spine: State of the Art Reviews 2:533–716, 1988. Philadelphia, Hanley & Belfus, Inc.

Chapter 3

DIAGNOSTIC EVALUATION

Richard B. Birrer, M.D., and
Michael P. DellaCorte, D.P.M.

THE LABORATORY EXAMINATION

As with all areas of clinical medicine, laboratory tests to evaluate and manage foot problems are supplementary. With few exceptions, laboratory data should not be routinely ordered. A complete blood count should not be ordered for screening purposes unless it forms a portion of a preoperative evaluation. Conversely, a urinalysis would be appropriate if there were suspicion of underlying diabetic or renal disease. Hematocrit should be tested if the feet are cold or cyanotic or if an anemia or polycythemia is suspected. The hemoglobin level can confirm these findings as well as other diverse conditions—for example, pernicious anemia, leukemia, and dietary and hereditary anemias. If an underlying infection is suspected, a white cell count with differential is appropriate. Rarely, leukemia may be discovered by noting undifferentiated cells in the white cell count. A VDRL (veneral disease research laboratory) test should be considered in the differential diagnosis of syphilitic-appearing dermopathy and unexplained ulcers and neuropathies. The erythrocyte sedimentation rate is of limited usefulness except in following the progress of patients with rheumatoid arthritis and in differentiating psychogenic from organic foot pain.

Of the numerous tests available, one must be selective in choosing, when there is clinical suspicion of underlying disease. For example, serum glucose is useful for following a diabetic's progress; serum urate would be warranted in a gout patient. The clinical diagnosis of xanthoma should prompt determination of the patient's lipid profile (cholesterol, triglycerides, lipoprotein electrophoresis). Finally, the physician should consider thyroid function tests if there is evidence of pretibial myxedema and hyperhidrosis (hyperthyroidism) or coarse nails and dry skin and hair of the foot (hypothyroidism).

Doppler studies of the feet and legs are recommended on suspicion of blood supply impairment. Electromyography is reserved for suspected neuromuscular or neurologic disorders; it is useful in the diagnosis of compartment syndromes. Scrapings, cultures, and biopsies may be necessary for diagnosing a wide variety of infectious and noninfectious conditions.

THE RADIOLOGIC EXAMINATION

Routine anteroposterior films of the foot do not demonstrate all areas satisfactorily due to nonconformity in thickness between the rearfoot and forefoot. Similarly, lateral x-rays are not informative at the level of the digits and metatarsals due to overlap. If the ankle is to be visualized also, it should be radiographed separately; conversely, ankle films will not visualize the foot well. Therefore, x-ray evaluation of the foot should be taken after a clinical impression or differential diagnosis has been established. Routine films of the foot are usually unwarranted, although they may occasionally reveal an unexpected asymptomatic pathologic problem. In general, views of specific areas should be taken or requested, and it is advisable for the purpose of diagnostic accuracy that radiographs of the normal side be taken for comparison.

23

The following x-ray views are the most commonly used in standard x-ray evaluation. Each shows different aspects of the bony anatomy of the foot.

Dorsoplantar (Anteroposterior) Projection

The dorsoplantar projection allows for evaluation and examination of transverse plane deformities of the foot involving the phalanges, metatarsals, tarsometatarsal joints, and navicular, cuboid, and cuneiforms. Normal values of the angles between the metatarsals and the phalanges have been established.

Technique. The patient is asked to place the foot on the x-ray plate. (It is essential to have the patient bear weight for a standard orthopedic evaluation of the foot. Weight bearing is not necessary in traumatic conditions.) The x-ray beam is then angled 15 degrees from the vertical to place the beam perpendicular to the metatarsals. The center of the beam is aimed at the lateral portion of the navicular. Both feet may be taken at one time, provided the plate is large enough, thus decreasing the patient's exposure to radiation.

Weight-bearing Lateral Projection

This lateral view is important in evaluating flatfoot and cavus foot deformities, dorsal and plantar exostosis, heel spurs, location of a foreign body, and assessment of the talus, calcaneus, and subtalar joint. The navicular, cuneiforms, metatarsals, and digits are views with overlap. Numerous angles have been developed to assist in surgical management of foot deformities.

Technique. The weight-bearing lateral view is taken with the aid of an orthoposer— a stand that holds the x-ray cassette vertical. The patient stands on the orthoposer and places the medial aspect of the affected foot against the cassette. The central beam of the x-ray is then aimed at the cuboid bone. Non-weight-bearing laterals are used in trauma.

Lateral Oblique Projection

The lateral oblique view is a non-weight-bearing supinated view of the foot. Supination of the foot causes overlap of bony structures to allow evaluation of the dorsolateral and plantar medial aspects of the foot only. It is used in trauma evaluation and as part of a complete foot x-ray series (dorsoplantar, lateral, medial oblique, and lateral oblique).

Technique. There are two methods of taking this film. In one, the foot is placed flat on the plate, and the x-ray beam is angled 45 degrees to the medial side of the foot and aimed at the cuboid bone. The second method places the x-ray beam in front of the foot at 15 degrees to the vertical. The foot is then rolled on the lateral side, bringing the medial aspect 45 degrees from the plate. The central beam is aimed at the cuboid bone.

Medial Oblique Projection

This non-weight-bearing view opens up the joints of the foot by pronation, allowing intra-articular evaluation. It is often used for evaluating forefoot trauma.

Technique. There are two methods of taking this view. In the first, the foot is placed flat on the plate, as for the dorsoplantar view. The x-ray beam is angled 45 degrees, aimed at the navicular bone, and positioned on the lateral aspect of the foot. The second method places the x-ray unit exactly as for a dorsoplantar view (angled at 15 degrees to vertical directly in front of the foot). The foot is placed on the plate, and the patient is asked to roll it on the medial side so that the lateral aspect is lifted 45 degrees from the plate.

Specific anteroposterior films are recommended for toes and metatarsophalangeal joints. A sesamoid view should be ordered of the sesamoid and metatarsal heads and is best achieved by having the patient passively dorsiflex a toe or foot with an elastic bandage or piece of muslin.

The medial oblique view is best for determining pathology of the lateral talus and the calcaneonavicular and fractures of the anterosuperior tubercle of the os calcis. Lateral and tangential radiographs (Harris view) are recommended for visualization of the os calcis. They should be slightly overexposed. A lead marker should be utilized for accurate localization of any underlying bony pathology or bony landmark.

Routine ankle x-rays comprise anterior, posterior, lateral, and oblique mortise films. Routine films should be supplemented by passive stress test radiographs when appropriate. Depending on the associated amount of spasm and pain, it may be necessary to use local regional (i.e., peroneal) or general anesthesia. If the stress films are positive, further evaluation is unnecessary. If stress films are inconclusive and there is strong clinical suspicion of a complete tear, an arthrogram should be ordered. After sterile preparation and drape, the test is performed on the anterior portion of the joint opposite the area of suspected injury. After initial aspiration, a 10-ml solution consisting of 1 ml lidocaine and 9 ml of contrast material (e.g., 25% Hypaque solution) is slowly injected; then anteroposterior, lateral, and oblique films are obtained. Although the dye may enter the tendon sheaths surrounding the ankle and may even flow to the subtalar joint, dye appearing outside the joint capsule or the surrounding tendon sheath is abnormal. The incidence of false-negative examinations rises significantly because of healing during the first week after injury. Arthroscopy can also help to detect tears and debris.

COMPUTERIZED TOMOGRAPHY (CT) AND MAGNETIC RESONANCE IMAGING (MRI)

CT and MRI are noninvasive techniques the produce soft tissue definition that cannot be achieved by conventional x-rays or nuclear scintigraphy. CT is excellent for assessing cortical bone. MRI is superior to CT for muscle, ligament, tendon, and cartilage elements due to its high resolution, superior soft tissue contrast, direct multiplanar imaging, and lack of ionizing radiation. MRI sensitivity in detecting focal areas of pathology and effusions is superior to CT and makes it the method of choice when imaging of the foot and ankle is indicated.

PHOTOGRAPHY

The primary care practitioner may want to photograph foot pathology for medical, legal, research, or teaching purposes. The following guidelines are recommended.

1. In general, photograph with maximum magnification only the area involved, unless the etiology (e.g., pes planus, tight shoe) is evident, which should then be included.

2. Take different views of the pathologic area.

3. If surgery is contemplated, take preoperative and postoperative clinical pictures.

4. A 35-mm camera with a behind-the-lens meter is the most practical and is generally sufficient.

5. A close-up lens (1+–10+ diopters) or macro lens (50–90 mm), though not necessary, will allow close, detailed photos without contamination of the surgical field.

6. Color film (ASA 100–400) is generally recommended for most office work. Speeds of less than 100 often require additional lighting or strobe, but the color is better and the grain finer. Black-and-white film (ASA 100–400) is suitable for many deformities. A matte white is best for dark-skinned patients and a matte black for light-skinned individuals. The speed will need to be decreased by one or two stops with matte white and increased one stop with matte black.

BIBLIOGRAPHY

1. Kingston S: Magnetic resonance imaging of the ankle and foot. Clin Sports Med 7:15–28, 1988.
2. Oloff-Solomon J, et al: Computed tomographic scanning of the foot and ankle. Clin Podiatr Med Surg 5:931–944, 1988.
3. Weissman S: Standard foot radiographic techniques for the foot and ankle. Clin Podiatr Med Surg 5:767–775, 1988.

Chapter 4

SKIN

Richard B. Birrer, M.D.

ANATOMY

The skin of the sole and the skin of the dorsum of the foot are anatomically distinct, which is an important fact in differentiating the features of their respective pathologies. The skin of the dorsum of the foot has a normal stratum corneum, but the skin of the sole of the foot is very thick. The next layer, the stratum lucidum, is present on the sole but is absent from the dorsal aspect of the foot. There are no hair follicles or sebaceous glands on the sole of the foot, but both are present in normal distribution on the dorsum. However, the eccrine glands are numerous on the sole, although there is a normal complement on the instep.

EXAMINATION

In addition to the routine skin exam (see Chapter 2) a Wood's light and biopsy may be useful. A Wood's (or black) light consists of ultraviolet long-wave light from a high-pressure mercury lamp fitted with a special nickel oxide and silica filter. All web spaces should be examined with light for fluorescein, particularly the coral red color characteristic of the diphtheroid-causing erythrasma. However, a variety of dyes, ointments, and debris may fluoresce various colors and lead to false diagnoses. Biopsy technique of the dorsum of the foot is similar to that of other areas of the body. A 1% lidocaine solution is used as a local anesthetic, and then an appropriate-sized cylindrical punch ranging from 2–10 mm is chosen. A rhythmic, alternating, clockwise-counterclockwise motion is made rapidly, and

a small surgical scissors is used to clip the biopsy plug from the underlying fat of the deep dermis. Bleeding can easily be controlled by application of basic ferric sulfate or subsulfate solution (Monsel's). A smaller punch is used when cosmesis is important, whereas a scalpel with an elliptical biopsy may be more appropriate if a larger specimen is needed. Biopsies of the sole of the foot, especially weight-bearing areas, must be done with the utmost caution in order to avoid development of painful scar tissue. The recommended size is 2–3 mm with 4–5 mm considered the maximum.

CONTACT DERMATITIS

Contact dermatitis can be classified as either allergic or secondary to irritating chemicals (Fig. 1). Pathologically, both types are characterized by a nonspecific, eczematous reaction with variable amounts of edema, erythema, vesicles, and occasionally bullae. Exposure to the rhus family (poison ivy, oak, or sumac) is a common cause of contact dermatitis, and the lesions tend to be linear and geographic in distribution, corresponding to area of contact. Another common cause of contact dermatitis is shoe wear. The dorsal aspects of the foot, particularly the hallux and distal portions, are usually involved. The reaction is due to the rubber found in the toe box of most shoes or the cement used to bind together certain shoe components. Leather is usually nonallergenic. In rare cases, the sole of the foot and other portions of the body may become involved in an id reaction. Pruritus is common.

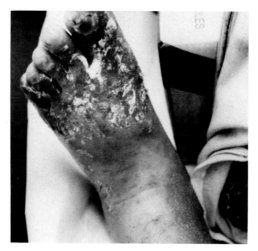

FIGURE 1. Contact dermatitis caused by new synthetic shoes.

Examples of primary irritant contact dermatitis include inadequately prepared chemical solutions, such as permanganate and Burow's; irritating creams; hot water; and highly concentrated chemical solutions. Individuals who have underlying systemic diseases, such as vasculitis, or diabetes, or peripheral vascular disease can develop severe contact dermatitis using over-the-counter callus and corn remedies. Occasionally, the dermatitis may be iatrogenically induced from a prescribed orthotic or similar device.

Diagnosis of contact dermatitis is determined by obtaining a careful history and an appropriate series of patch tests. The patch test is more easily administered by serial dilution of the suspected agent(s) and their application by Band-Aids or a similar device to the upper back for 48–72 hours. A control should also be applied and the area examined every 24 hours with the results carefully documented. It is important to dilute and prepare the topical agents adequately according to a number of readily available tablets for patch tests and preparations. Inadequately diluted agents produce edema, erythema, and vesicles of an irritant nature in the majority of healthy individuals. A well-demarcated, unnatural outline to a patch test suggests contact sensitivity.

The treatment of choice is twofold. First, the offending agent must be removed. Usually, substitution of a leather upper is sufficient, although in some individuals substitution of a thermoplastic or Silastic toe box for a rubber one is necessary. The additional prescription of a regularly applied drying powder together with cotton or woolen socks rather than synthetic ones will increase aeration and thus reduce the solvent effect of perspiration on allergens in the shoes. Second, in mild to moderate cases, a topical steroid such as hydrocortisone or triamcinolone is sufficient. In severe cases, a more potent topical steroid (e.g., betamethasone) in combination with a systemic steroid regimen for several days may be required.

ECCRINE GLAND DISORDERS

Hyperhidrosis

Hyperhidrosis is an annoying condition that frequently affects the palms and soles, particularly when tension and safety are high. It may be worse when accompanied by an offending odor (i.e., bromhidrosis). Hyperhidrosis is usually idiopathic, though it is important to rule out certain diseases that can aggravate or cause the condition: thyrotoxicosis, palmar and plantar keratoses, cholinergic medications, and fever from any cause, particularly the night sweats of lymphoma and tuberculosis, pheochromocytoma, gout, and carcinoid syndrome. Because of the warm, moist environment usually associated with plantar hyperhidrosis, warts and tinea pedis often develop.

Treatment of the condition is frequently frustrating. Locally, a diluted formalin or glutaraldehyde solution (3–10%) may be useful, although there may be some discoloration and possible allergic sensitization in the susceptible individual. A mild solution of potassium permanganate (1%) is more effective if bromhidrosis is a problem. Topically drying powders (Zea Sorb) applied at bedtime and occluded with a thin plastic film such as Saran Wrap are helpful, though far from curative. If bromhidrosis is a major problem, antiseptic soaps or solutions in combination with an antiperspirant can result in improvement. The combination of equal amounts of baking soda and talc applied twice daily may also be beneficial. The patient should be advised to reduce intake of spicy foods such as onions and garlic. Finally, for both conditions, the wearing of nonocclusive, nonsynthetic socks and leather footwear is essential for maximal aeration of the feet. In rare cases, systemic agents such as anticholinergic drugs and anxiolytic tranquilizers can be used with some benefits.

Dyshidrosis

An eczematous disease of the epidermis, dyshidrosis, is characterized by numerous yellow, deep-seated vesicles that affect the soles and the palms in its acute stage. The condition, also termed pompholyx, is often accompanied by hyperhidrosis and pruritus. Scaling and erythematous macules and papules denote the healing phase. The differential diagnosis should consider pustular psoriasis, tinea pedis of the plantar vesicular type, epidermolysis bullosa, and keratolysis exfoliative. The recommended management consists of wet soaks with saline or Burow's solution (i.e., aluminum acetate) followed by the application of a topical steroid. Severe or refractory cases might benefit from administration of a systemic steroid. Recurrences are common.

FUNGAL INFECTIONS

Tinea pedis (i.e., athlete's foot) is the most common dermatophytosis in the United States. It may be a relatively minor chronic infection, or it may cause a disabling dermatitis characterized by large blisters, fissures, thickening of the sole, and secondary infection. The most common causes are *Trichophyton rubrum* and *Trichophyton mentagrophytes*, although clinical presentation varies:

1. Dry type (i.e., moccasin type), usually of the toe web spaces or the sole and heel of the foot, is associated with varying amounts of scaling, erythemia, pruritus, and fissuring.

2. Wet type is of either the sole of the foot or the web spaces (Fig. 2).

3. A dermatophytic or vesicular variety marked by a profound amount of inflammation may involve the palms and fingers.

The differential diagnosis should include either erythrasma (Wood's light), soft corn, psoriasis, keratoses, and contact dermatitis in the dry form or epidermolysis bullosa, pustular psoriasis, and dyshidrosis in the wet form or the vesicular form of tinea pedis.

A fungal infection of the foot is diagnosed by microscopic examination of suspected material scraped from the margin of the diseased area or a vesicle wall (not its contents) with a No. 15 scalpel blade. The material is then gently heated with a few drops of 10% potassium hydroxide solution, and a coverslip is applied. Branching hyphae and myceliae are diagnostic of superficial dermatophytes. Budding cells and pseudohyphae are suggestive of

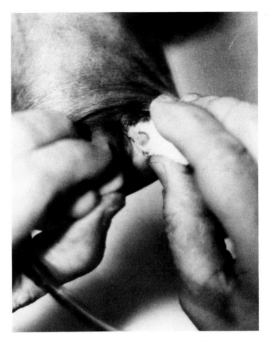

FIGURE 2.   Fungal infection of web space.

yeast, particularly monilia. When the test is negative or nonconfirmatory, some of the suspected material should be planted on a suitable culture medium such as Sabouraud's agar. The tops of the bottles should be loose to provide sufficient aeration; at least 2 weeks in a dark, warm environment should be allowed for full growth to occur. The diagnostic accuracy of red color change for identification of dermatophytes is over 95% within 14 days. If fluffy white colonies are also present, the diagnostic accuracy exceeds 97%.

The dry forms of tinea pedis usually respond well to antifungal solutions and creams applied at bedtime and in the morning (Table 1). A mild keratolytic agent such as salicylic acid (Whitfield's ointment) or a coal tar preparation (Pragmatar) is a useful supplement for the dry, diffuse plantar type associated with variable degrees of keratosis. Griseofulvin ultramicrosize (Fulvicin P/G, Grisactin Ultra, Gris-PEG, or Grifulvin V [children] 500–1,000 mg daily for a month) may be useful for the refractory dry, interdigital type or the diffuse plantar form. The agent is well tolerated, and side effects are minimal. Many experts do not consider hematologic or hepatic monitoring necessary. Recalcitrant infections can be treated with oral ketoconazole 200 mg/day; however, liver function must be monitored due to risk of hepatotoxicity. Vesicular and dermatophytic

TABLE 1. *Topical Antifungal Medications*

Name	Doses per Day	Efficacy	Comments
Undecylenic acid and derivatives	As needed	++	Antibacterial/antifungal—tinea pedis, cruris, corporis, versicolor
Iodochlorhydroxyquin 3%	2 or 3 (no more than 1 week)	+	Stains skin, clothing; interferes with thyroid function tests
Triacetin	2	+	Broad-spectrum antifungal
Haloprogin 1%	2	+++	Broad-spectrum antifungal
Tolnaftate 1%	2	+	Broad-spectrum antifungal
Nystatin 100,000 units/gm	2 or 3	+++	Antifungal activity mainly for Candida
Amphotericin 3%	2–4	++	Antifungal activity mainly for Candida
Gentian Violet 1%	2–4	+	Antibacterial, gram-positive/antifungal; cannot apply to ulcerative lesion; stains and tattoos skin
Imidazole Agents of Choice			
Miconazole 2% (Micatin, Monistat-Derm)	2	++++	Broad-spectrum antifungal—tinea pedis, cruris, corporis, and vesicular Candida—not used in children (< 2 yrs)
Econazole 1% (Spectazole)	2	++++	Broad-spectrum antifungal—tinea pedis, cruris, corporis, and versicolor
Ciclopirox olamine 1% (Loprox)	2	++++	Broad-spectrum antifungal
Clotrimazole 1% Lotrimin, Mycelex)	2	++++	Broad-spectrum antifungal
Oxiconazole 1% (Oxistat)	2	++++	Broad-spectrum antifungal
Sulconazole 11% (Exelderm)	2	++++	Broad-spectrum antifungal with gram-positive antibacterial activity
Ketoconazole 2% (Nizoral)	1	++++	Broad-spectrum antifungal
Naftifine hydrochloride 1% (Naftin)	2	++++	Broad-spectrum antifungal

forms of tinea pedis respond well to the application of wet soaks (potassium permanganate 1:10,000, silver nitrate 1:200, or Burow's solution 1:20) initially until the skin returns to normal; then they should be discontinued. Prolonged application of wet soaks can result in extreme desiccation, cracking, and fissuring, particularly of the surrounding normal skin. A systemic antibiotic such as erythromycin or tetracycline may be required if there is a secondary bacterial infection. If the inflammation and vesiculation are severe, 40–60 mg daily of prednisone followed by a 5-mg reduction every 2–3 days depending on response is quite helpful. Once the acute inflammatory response has subsided, oral griseofulvin or a topical antifungal agent in combination with a steroid cream can complete the therapy. If the palmar surface of the hands is also involved, it need not be actively treated other than with application of wet dressings, because the skin will return to normal after resolution of the pedal disease.

Finally, the patient should be carefully educated about adequate aeration of the feet through the use of nonocclusive, nonsynthetic socks and footwear and the use of open shoes (e.g., sandals). A mild antifungal powder can be applied in the morning, particularly in the web spaces, as a precaution, and is especially recommended in the humid and warm months of the year and before exercising. The patient should be reminded that recurrences are common, particularly in susceptible individuals.

WARTS

Viral warts—verrucae vulgaris—are common on the plantar surface of the feet (Fig. 3). They usually present as white, firm, small growths but can appear as flat lesions on the sole or be exuberant or cauliflowerlike in other locations of the foot. Warts are caused by the papovavirus, with the average life expectancy of a clone of virions being anywhere from 4–9 months. Spontaneous regression is, therefore, common. A number of small warty masses may coalesce, forming larger mosaic warts. Patients who usually develop warts do not have a history of trauma, though they may have a history of warts elsewhere on the body. Warts may be asymptomatic or cause severe

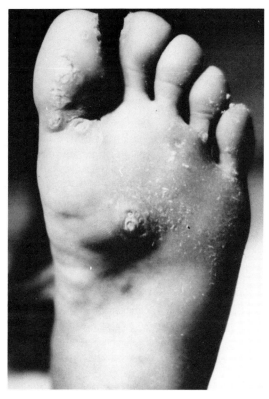

FIGURE 3. Multiple plantar warts.

to define its borders. Thereafter, an electrocautery needle is placed in the central superficial portion and the unit activated for a few seconds until the wart "boils." A small curette can then be used to remove the necrotic tissue; attempts to remove deeper tissue should be avoided, because scarring will result. Because verrucal growth is superficial, more effort should be spent on its lateral margins, since that is the area where recurrence is most likely. Hand pressure with a gauze pad after application of ferric subsulfate (Monsel's solution) is sufficient to stop most bleeding. The wound should then be packed with an antibiotic ointment (e.g., Ilotycin, Neosporin, Bacitracin), and a horseshoe-shaped adhesive felt pad applied to disperse weight-bearing pressure (Fig. 4). The same techniques can be used if excisional therapy with a No. 15 scalpel blade is chosen. Once again, it is imperative not to invade the deeper tissue of the dermis, but rather to use light electrocautery and curettage to remove any remaining tissue.

Biweekly application of liquid nitrogen is usually received more favorably by patients. Although this technique is not as effective as excisional surgery or electrosurgery, it is far less painful. The more radical modalities

pain and disability if they are present over sensitive weight-bearing areas of the foot. Warts tend to interrupt the normal papillary skin lines and produce pinpoint capillary bleeding when pared with a scalpel blade. Lateral compression causes pain. The differential diagnosis would include hyperkeratotic plantar lesions such as corns and calluses, foreign body reactions, fibromas, and the unusual lesion termed porokeratosis plantaris descreta, which is characterized by severe pain and the absence of pinpoint bleeding.

Treatment is tailored to the type and location of the wart. Large plantar warts, particularly the asymptomatic mosaic variety, should be treated conservatively with weekly paring and the application of a keratolytic agent such as 40% salicylic acid plaster, 50% trichloroacetic acid, and lactic acids. Such treatment modalities suffice for the majority of asymptomatic plantar warts. More invasive techniques (e.g., electrosurgery, cryotherapy, excisional surgery, laser) should be reserved for painful lesions. After a local lidocaine (1%) anesthetic block with 1:100,000 epinephrine (avoiding epinephrine in the digits), the lesion is pared carefully

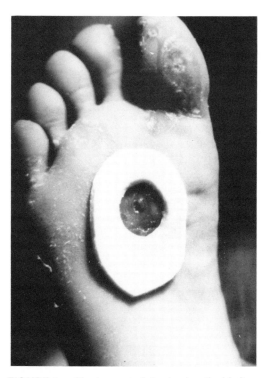

FIGURE 4. Plantar warts following two liquid nitrogen applications and a protective donut.

should be reserved for removal of a large "mother" wart, which will then cause regression of "baby" satellite warts. Rarely, radiotherapy for recalcitrant plantar warts can be employed but only in consultation with an experienced operator.

Periungual or subungual warts are not uncommon. They often deform the nail plate and may, if deep enough, erode the underlying bony tuft. These lesions are best managed by conservative surgical removal following anesthetic nerve block. Blunt dissection or curettage is preferred over electrosurgery or the scalpel. Electrodesiccation or laser can be used to remove any remaining warty tissue, and Monsel's solution is preferred to electrosurgery for control of bleeding.

CALLUSES/TYLOMATA

A callus is a more diffuse, hyperkeratotic lesion that, like a corn, develops in response to pressure irritation and friction (Fig. 5). Usually the sites of tylomata are the ball of the foot, a protuberant bony enlargement, or the

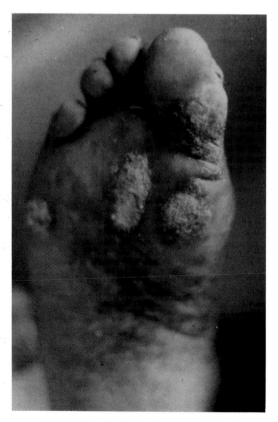

FIGURE 5. Multiple plantar callosities.

area of an abnormal weight distribution (i.e., lateral border of the foot and the fifth toe, below the metatarsal heads, or the perimeter of the heel, particularly the medial portion). Less common sites include the talar head, the prominent navicular tuberosity, the dorsal surface of the first metatarsal cuneiform joint, the medial portion of the first metatarsal phalangeal joint over a hallux abducto valgus, and certain unusual areas in association with such congenital anomalies as clubfoot or claw foot.

The lesion is diffuse and therefore does not have clearly demonstrated margins such as helomata. Initially, the area is erythematous, but in time a yellowish-gray, slightly raised hyperkeratotic region is formed, which preserves the papillary skin lines. It is often diffusely tender when direct pressure is applied. Conservative treatment includes periodic paring with a scalpel blade (i.e., weekly to monthly) and the application of an adhesive felt, latex, or foam rubber protective donut or horseshoe (see Chapter 20). Keratolytic agents such as 20–40% salicylic acid and plaster can be applied for several days every week over several weeks.

As with corns, it is essential to treat the underlying etiology responsible for the stress (e.g., deformity, disease, biomechanical dysfunction). In the female, high-heeled shoes are often responsible for placing increased amounts of pressure on the metatarsal heads or the bases of the phalanges. A tight toe box forces the toes backward as well as together, particularly at the metatarsophalangeal joints. In the malfunctioning foot, a flexible sole will aggravate abnormal stress. Shoes that are too narrow or that place frictional forces on the medial and lateral borders, particularly where the seams meet at the upper and the insole, must be modified. Even elastic stockings can increase frictional forces on the ball of the foot, pulling the toes backward. Abnormal gait due to hyperpronated feet or genu valgus or varus deformity of the knees may also produce pronounced stresses on certain areas of the feet. Finally, local pedal conditions such as bursitis, tenosynovitis, tumors, spurs, exostosis, and osteophytes often can lead to or aggravate existing calluses. Therefore, effective management of the patient with tylomata consists of treating the underlying etiology.

CORNS/HELOMATA

Helomata have been classified into two types: dura (hard) and molle (soft) (Fig. 6). A

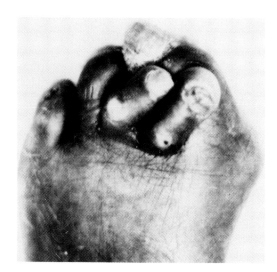

FIGURE 6. Helomata of the dorsal second and third toes in association with overlap and hallux valgus.

corn is a focal hyperkeratotic lesion secondary to pressure or irritation from an external (e.g., shoe) or internal (e.g., exostosis, unreduced dislocation, hypertrophic phalangeal condyle) source. The most common sites for hard corns are the dorsal aspects of the lesser toes of the proximal or interphalangeal level and the lateral region of the fifth toe. If there is a flexion or mallet toe deformity, the terminal end of the small toes may develop an end corn. Over time, due to repeated microirritation, an inflammatory reaction occurs with a buildup of cellular debris and compensatory epidermal hyperplasia. There is no age limit to corns; children have developed them. Corns may or may not be painful, though direct pressure over the lesion usually produces variable amounts of discomfort. Unlike warts, corns do not bleed when pared by a scalpel blade. They appear as a thickened epidermal area with a conical center that is lighter in color than the overlying epidermis. The epidermal lines are interrupted, unlike a callus, which preserves the lines.

The differential diagnosis of hard corns should include verrucae—distinguished by their disruption of the papillary skin lines, capillary bleeding on surgical paring, and pain on lateral compression—foreign bodies, and fibromas.

Soft corns usually appear between the toes and result from the irritative pressure of one condyle rubbing against its neighbor due to the differential lengths of the toes and metatarsals. Macerated skin, usually associated with soft corns in a toe web space, often resembles a fungal infection. The treatment of a misdiagnosed soft corn with ointments, creams, and other chemical substances usually aggravates the lesion and may produce such complications as fissuring, further skin irritation, and fibrosis.

The treatment of corns is twofold: conservative and surgical. The conservative method of treatment consists of periodic, weekly to monthly paring of the hyperkeratotic area with a No. 15 scalpel blade. The paring procedure is done in short, rhythmical, crescentic movements until the overlying epidermis is removed and the softer portions of the underlying corn are visible. Specially tailored, adhesive-backed felt pads in the shape of a horseshoe or donut are then fitted to the area to allow pressure dispersion to nonaffected areas. Specially fitted foam or latex pads can also be used, depending on the preference of the practitioner. For soft corns, lamb's wool pads can be placed between the affected toes.

Shoe wear should be carefully examined and modified in order to reduce frictional pressures. If the shoe is leather, a special device called a shoemaker's swan can be used to stretch the area causing the irritation. An alternative shoe may, of necessity, need to be prescribed for the healing phase.

Surgical excision of the lesions should be reserved for the most refractory cases after a 6-month trial of conservative therapy and in particular should be decided with the utmost discretion in the foot at risk (i.e., in the patient with diabetes or peripheral vascular disease).

Surgical therapy should be handled in consultation with a podiatrist or orthopedic surgeon. Local excision of hard and soft corns without simultaneous removal of the irritative focus (e.g., poorly fitted shoe, protuberant condyle, dislocated phalangeal joint) is not recommended, because recurrence will follow and complications such as fibrotic scarring and sinus tract development may result. The procedure can be performed in the outpatient department and under a local anesthetic nerve block. After a hemiphalangectomy or condylectomy, the wound is closed with sutures, and a dry, sterile dressing is applied. Children and the elderly are best managed conservatively.

An end corn is managed similarly to corns in other areas; the treatment of choice is conservative and palliative. Moleskin, foam rubber, or latex is applied to the toe so that the distal end of the toe is protected. The nail is also trimmed to reduce impingement. If there is abnormal flexion of the distal interphalangeal joint, with or without fixed skeletal deformity (e.g., mallet toe or clawtoe deformity), it should be corrected (see Chapters 7 and 20).

MISCELLANEOUS KERATOSES

A number of other keratotic lesions afflict the foot, which by definition are not caused by friction and are frequently hereditary. Keratoses affecting the soles of the feet usually afflict the palms of the hands simultaneously. From the perspective of the primary care physician, these conditions should form part of the routine differential diagnosis of plantar keratotic lesions. Examples of punctate keratoses include those inherited dominantly and recessively. Secondary syphilis, arsenic poisoning, Darier's disease, and basal cell nevus syndrome may be associated with this form of keratosis. Differential diagnosis should also include guttate psoriasis. More diffuse forms of keratosis may be genetic, as in the dominant form of Unna-Thost disease, or be associated with such skin diseases as psoriasis, pityriasis, rosacea, lichen planus, syphilis, or pityriasis rubra pilaris. Furthermore, noninherited diffuse keratosis may, in a small number of cases, be a harbinger of internal malignancy.

The treatment of these lesions is frustrating due to rapid regrowth of skin. Frequent paring and the use of keratolytic agents (e.g., salicylic acid) and, more recently, retinoic acid preparations have been applied with some success.

INFECTIOUS DISEASES

Scabies

The web spaces of the toes are often affected by the itch mite *Sarcoptes scabiei*, though less commonly than the hands. The patient usually complains of itching, which is especially bad at night. The diagnosis of scabies is made by a suggestive history and the observation of papulovesicles, nondescript papules, and identification of the characteristic burrow, which is a very thin, narrow, serpiginous track in which the egg-laying female mite resides. Identification of the mite in the skin scrapings or, more rarely, in a biopsy is confirmatory. It is also important to check the patient's torso, particularly in the bathing suit area, and genitalia. The differential diagnosis should include tinea pedis, contact dermatitis, and dyshidrosis.

Therapy consists of treating the patient and the patient's contacts with one or two applications of 1% lindane (Kwell) or crotamiton solution (Eurax). It is important to advise the patient that it may be several weeks to months until the pruritus, probably an immunologic phenomenon, subsides.

Bacterial Infections

The elaboration of keratolytic enzyme by a diphtheroid bacteria produces multiple small, superficial pits that are rapidly filled with debris. The condition, termed pitted keratolysis, may produce some discomfort, slight pruritus, and characteristic dark punctate lesions of the heel. Diagnosis is confirmed by bacterial culture, although clinical observation is usually sufficient. Treatment consists of the application of erythromycin ointment or systemic erythromycin, 400 mg twice daily for 2 weeks.

Streptococcus can follow fungal infections, especially if cracks and fissures develop between the web spaces of the toes. If early cellulitis and localized infection are not aggressively treated, recurrent bouts of lymphangitis and erysipelas can present varying degrees of elephantiasis. The treatment of choice is systemic penicillin given orally.

Impetigo contagiosa, secondary to staphylococci or streptococci, can also affect the feet, particularly if the epidermal barrier has been violated by previous fungal or vesicular disease. Papules with honey-colored crusts are characteristic. Penicillin or erythromycin by mouth is curative.

Gram-negative bacteria can also superinfect previously inflamed and injured areas of the foot, especially in the immunocompromised host. Characteristically, the erosions may suggest tinea pedis, but cultures and scrapings are negative. Diagnosis is made by smear and bacterial culture, and treatment consists of an astringent soak (e.g., silver nitrate 0.5% Burow's solution) and an effective systemic antibiotic.

FOREIGN BODIES

Foreign bodies in the plantar surface of the foot are not infrequent, particularly among shoeless individuals. Such foreign bodies often enter the foot without the patient being aware of it. Splinters are the most common foreign objects, although hairs, pebbles, glass, and gunshot pellets are also found. If a foreign body is suspected, an x-ray should be taken to localize it. Most types of glass are radiopaque. The differential diagnosis should include corns, verrucae, and such miscellaneous conditions as pyogenicum granuloma and fibroma. For superficial foreign bodies, the lesions should be gently pared, and a curette and splinter forceps used to remove the object. Such management is usually curative, but wet dressings and a topical antibiotic may be helpful. Rarely, if there is secondary cellulitis or lymphangitis, a systemic antibiotic should be used. For deeper foreign bodies, surgical management is discussed in Chapter 13.

ATOPIC DERMATITIS

The feet can be involved in atopic dermatitis or eczema, particularly in patients with an allergic diathesis—asthma, hay fever, and so on. Acute pedal manifestations of the dermatoses include erythema, edema, warmth, and pain. Chronically, there are both scaling and lichenification. There may be fissuring and maceration of the toe web spaces following secondary infection. The differential diagnosis should include contact dermatitis and tinea pedis. Patch testing will be positive in the former condition, and scrapings and culture are confirmatory in the latter. Furthermore, atopic dermatitis does not typically involve the web spaces. Treatment consists of the application of a steroid cream once or twice daily. Mild cases and those requiring long-term use are best handled by using 0.5%, 1%, or 2.5% hydrocortisone. More severe acute cases are handled with one of the newer fluorinated steroids (e.g., betamethasone). If the skin is dry and scaly, an ointment is preferred, whereas a normally hydrated skin cream may be useful. For macerated, eczematous lesions, lotions are more suitable. Use of a thin plastic film at night improves the penetrating effect of topical ointment on dry skin. In severe cases, systemic prednisone with a several-week taper is necessary. Antipruritic agents such as cyproheptadine or diphenhydramine may be necessary to break the itch-inflammation cycle. Soaps, detergents, and other drying agents are best avoided during the acute phase. Nonsynthetic loose stockings and socks should be worn.

PSORIASIS

This condition is a dominantly inherited disorder characterized by reddish-pink papules and plaques of silver-gray scales. The areas affected usually involve the scalp, knees, lumbosacral area, elbows, and penis, although there are more generalized forms of the eruption over the whole body. There may be variable degrees of pruritus and associated pitting of the nails as well as an erosive deforming arthritis. Psoriasis of the feet presents either as random scaly papules or plaques on the dorsal or plantar aspects of the foot or as hyperkeratotic plaques that are fissured in the area of the heel, pustular lesions of the sole, or macerated "white psoriasis" of the interdigital areas. The differential diagnosis should include lichen planus, atopic dermatitis, lupus erythematosus, and, in the macerated area, tinea pedis, soft corns, and moniliasis. The diagnosis of psoriasis is made by careful history and clinical exam, although appropriate fungal cultures may be necessary to rule out tinea pedis. Lesions usually respond well to application of steroid cream or ointment in conjunction with a keratolytic agent or tar and occlusive dressing such as a thin plastic film that will increase the absorption and effectiveness of these agents. Interdigital psoriasis is difficult to treat but usually responds well to intralesional steroid therapy (weekly injections of 0.1 ml of triamcinolone 10 mg/ml). No more than 1 mg of triamcinolone should be injected in any one area, because atrophy may result. Pustular psoriasis does not respond well to most therapeutic regimens; it should be handled in consultation with a specialist. It may be necessary both to administer periodic injections of triamcinolone (40 mg/ml) intramuscularly and to incise and drain the pustules. Further, antimetabolites as well as psoralen and ultraviolet-A (PUVA) may be necessary.

GRANULOMA ANNULARE

This lesion is a symptomatic idiopathic disease typically involving the dorsal surface of the feet. Children are more commonly affected than adults, and females twice as often as males. Diabetes mellitus should be suspected in the generalized form of the disease. The characteristic lesion is a donut-shaped ring of discrete pink papules. In time, these papules coalesce into annular plaques. The differential diagnosis should include lichen planus, erythema multiforme, larva migrans, and tinea pedis. Biopsy, which is usually not necessary, will be confirmatory. The natural history of granuloma annulare is spontaneous resolution in almost all cases; for those that are refractory or recurrent, intralesional injections of a steroid (e.g., triamcinolone) are useful.

MISCELLANEOUS CONDITIONS

The erythematous bull's-eye lesions of erythema multiforme may affect the feet. Diagnosis is made by noting the presence of the lesion in other areas of the body, including mucous membranes, as well as identifying the underlying predisposing conditions. The differential diagnosis should include tinea pedis, which can be documented by fungal culture and microscopic examination of the scrapings, and granuloma annulare. The pedal manifestations of erythema multiforme improve when the systemic disease is treated.

Epidermolysis bullosa is a vesiculobullous disease. Its presentation depends on a variety of hereditary factors, the presence or absence of fibrotic scarring, and the location of the split in the skin. Depending on the type, there are variable amounts of vesicles and bullae in association with erythema and hyperkeratosis. Diagnosis is made by a careful history, clinical exam, and biopsy. Immunofluorescent tests are usually negative. The differential diagnosis should include pustular psoriasis and dyshidrotic eczema. Of note is the fact that the noninherited acquired form of epidermolysis bullosa, which begins later in life, may be associated with underlying multiple myeloma, diabetes mellitus, or colitis. All forms of this disease respond to systemic steroids. Trauma should be avoided. Wet dressings and topical steroid creams are helpful. Chronic foot and toe contractions may develop, requiring correctional surgery and rehabilitation.

A number of autoimmune diseases can cause pedal dermopathy. In rare cases, the atrophic erythematous irregular plaques of discoid lupus erythematosus can involve the sole of the foot. Diagnosis is established by biopsy and by immunofluorescent and serologic tests. The differential diagnosis should include psoriasis and tinea pedis. Intralesional steroids accompanied by topical applications are helpful in resolving the plaques. Systemic lupus erythematosus may cause distal periungual redness of the toes. Gottron's sign, the appearance of glazed purplish-red coalescent papules forming plaques over the ankles and large toe, may be seen in patients with dermatomyositis. The usual skin changes associated with systemic scleroderma can be seen in the foot. When palpated, the skin is usually hard and blanched; chronically there may be ulceration and calcinosis of the heel. Finally, the "great mimicker," syphilis, should always be considered in any dermatologic condition involving the foot. Typically the skin lesions of secondary syphilis produce bilaterally symmetric, dry, reddish-brown macules, papules, pustules, or papulosquamous lesions. These syphilids are seldom pruritic and occasionally may involve the interdigital area and escape notice. A careful history and exam, accompanied by the appropriate serologic tests, will confirm the diagnosis. The differential diagnosis should include psoriasis, lichen planus, drug eruptions, pityriasis rosacea, and other acute exanthemata.

ULCERS

There are three basic ulcer types: neurotrophic/neuropathic, vascular/ischemic, and stasis/pressure (see Table 2, p. 77). Etiologies include diabetes, vascular disease, leprosy, cerebral palsy, alcoholism, and cord lesions such as spina bifida and syringomyelia. Their presentation and treatment are discussed in Chapter 11.

BIBLIOGRAPHY

1. Evanski PM, Reinherz RP: Easing the pain of common foot problems. Patient Care 25:38–53, 1991.
2. Parieser DM: Superficial fungal infections. Postgrad Med 87:205–214, 1990.
3. Silferskjöld JP: Common foot problems. Postgrad Med 89:183–188, 1991.

Chapter 5

NAILS

Richard B. Birrer, M.D.

ANATOMY

The nail, or unguis, is a horny elastic plate that covers the dorsal surface of the distal half of the terminal phalanx of each finger and toe. Histologically the nail consists of three layers: ventral, intermediate, and dorsal. The distal exposed portion, termed the nail body, is derived from the proximal hidden part, called the root. The nail wall, which is a fold of skin, surrounds the nail bed on each side. The nail groove is a slit between the wall and the bed. The eponychium is a proximal skin-fold covering about 25% of the nail and its root. The lunula is a white, semicircular area just distal to the eponychium. The nail plate grows longitudinally from the nail matrix. Finally, the paronychium represents the soft tissue surrounding the nail border.

It takes 4–6 months for a toenail to grow from its matrix to the free edge. Growth of the nail is continuous throughout life and averages 0.2–0.4 mm per week.

DYSTROPHIC NAILS (ONYCHODYSTROPHY)

Dystrophic nail is a general term representing the end-stage degenerative changes of the nail bed and plate (Fig. 1). The etiology may include poor hygiene, the aging process, trauma, or a variety of chronic diseases (e.g., hypothyroidism, diabetes). The nails are brownish-black in color and tend to be heaped up by cellular detritus, which fragments easily and has a waxy consistency. It is not clinically possible to distinguish dystrophic nails from fungal infections, although

the former tend to involve all the toes, whereas the latter involve only one or two adjacent ones. Culture and microscopic exams are essential. Treatment consists of careful paring of the nails with a clipper on a monthly basis and a review of nail hygiene. It is important to inform the patient that the nails will never return to their previous state.

ONYCHOMYCOSIS

Fungal infections of the toenails are not uncommon. They are particularly frustrating because of their chronic relapsing nature. They occur under or within the nail plate and cause a proliferation of keratinized debris under the nail. The nail thickens and crumbles when the plate is infected. Onychomycosis must be differentiated from nail dystrophy through microscopic examination and culture of the scrapings. Bacteria and candida, not dermatophytes, typically infect paronychial tissue. The treatment of onychomycosis is twofold. Conservatively, the nail should be periodically trimmed both in length and in depth. Shoe gear should be adequate, particularly the toe box, and socks should be nonsynthetic and loose. The use of topical antifungal agents is, for the most part, ineffective. The current treatment of choice is the use of micropulverized or microcrystalline griseofulvin in doses of 500–1,000 mg daily. Therapy must be continued for 1–2 years for a favorable response. The patient should be warned of common side effects such as headache, gastrointestinal discomfort, and occasionally photosensitivity and liver dysfunction. Laser waffling or surgical removal of the nail and matricectomy are

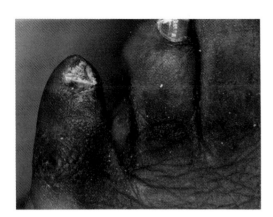

FIGURE 1.   Dystrophic nails.

reserved for refractory cases that serve as a nidus for infection in patients with diabetes or vascular disease (see Chapter 20).

SUBUNGUAL HEMATOMA

A traumatic blow to the nail can lead to a subungual hematoma. The individual is often immobilized due to throbbing pain as the blood tries to expand in the closed space. The severity of pain is proportional to the amount of trauma and pressure caused by the expanding hematoma. Ice should be applied immediately and the nail plate punctured to release the blood. Several methods are available. In the office, a dentist drill (or a laser in the pulse mode) is the fastest and least painful. A soldering gun with a fine point is also useful, although considerable expense can be saved by heating a paper clip or safety pin. On the field, a hand-held, battery-operated cautery gun can be used, as can a heated paper clip. Perhaps the best all-around modality in terms of expense and ease is gently rotating an 18-gauge needle through the plate. No anesthesia is necessary.

Once released, cold water soaks with gentle pressure will remove all the blood. A small, absorbent bandage is supplied, and nonsteroidal anti-inflammatory drugs or analgesics are prescribed for pain. The patient should be advised that the nail plate will be discolored by the hemoglobin pigments as it grows distally. If the blow was severe and the hematoma large, the nail may be lost entirely, although a new one will grow from the matrix in several months. Occasionally the matrix may be damaged during the trauma, resulting in a permanently deformed nail. X-rays should be taken to assess bone integrity.

INGROWN TOENAIL (UNGUIS INCARNATUS/ONYCHOCRYPTOSIS)

Although jokes about ingrown toenails abound, for the patient who has one it is far from being a laughing matter. A tight toe box or the congenital variation of tubular nails causes the nail plate to become curved rather than flat. The lateral (fibular) and medial (tibial) edges of the nail tend to become vertical, resembling an inverted C and impact on the horizontal bed of the nail. Usually the first toe is involved, although in some individuals any of the other toes may become similarly affected. In time, the leading edge of the curled toenail acts like a sharp foreign body, causing local inflammation and fungal or bacterial infection. A localized abscess with swelling and purulent discharge can occur. The abscess is frequently located on the lateral (fibular) side perhaps due to pressure against the second toe. With recurrent formation of small abscesses and inflammation, exuberant granulation tissue can form, thus creating a vicious cycle of inflammation, inadequate drainage, and enlargement of granulation tissue followed by fibrosis and further inhibition of drainage.

Treatment of the infection and the inflammation response consists of saucerization and removal of the ingrowing nail edge. If the lesion is mildly infected and has a minimal amount of granulation tissue, saucerization may be sufficient. A small amount of cotton is packed under the ingrown nail edge so that the skin is separated from the nail, thus allowing better drainage as well as preventing any further cutting action of the nail. If possible, without local anesthesia, the practitioner can trim away the ingrown part of the nail and instruct the patient to soak the toe three times a day in a solution of 1 tbsp Epsom salt and 1 tbsp povidone-iodine solution per pan of water. This conservative management suffices in the majority of mild to moderate lesions. If the lesion is exceptionally painful, a local anesthetic block may be necessary (see Chapter 20).

AVULSION OR PARTIAL AVULSION OF NAIL

Individuals who have chronically recurrent infections of ingrown toenails should be considered for complete and permanent removal of the nail. Consultation should be sought if the practitioner is unfamiliar or uncomfortable with the technique, because it is essential to remove the nail bed and matrix completely since small islands of nail tissue can reappear. A phenol, laser, or surgical matricectomy may be chosen.

Matricectomy

Removal of the nail matrix can follow partial or complete nail removal and may be done chemically, surgically, or by laser. The procedure is usually reserved for recurrent or refractory cases of ingrown toenails. There should be no infection present.

COMMON NAIL DEFORMITIES

The three most common nail deformities are tubular nails, hypertrophic thickening (onychophosis), and onychogryposis. The ram's horn deformity of onychogryposis most frequently involves the first toe but may also affect the small toes. Usually the nail plate is separated from the nail bed, is relatively brittle, and is seen in the elderly individual who is unable to trim the toenails. Treatment is conservative: trimming the nails. In younger individuals, excision of the matrix and the entire nail may be warranted.

Tubular nail deformity is usually congenital, although it may be exacerbated by a tight toe box. The inverted C becomes exaggerated and sometimes almost forms a complete circle (O). Treatment is identical to that for an ingrown toenail. Subungual exostosis, diagnosed by radiography, should be surgically removed.

More commonly seen in the middle-age and geriatric age groups, hypertrophic nail thickening is marked by considerable deformity and the deposition of discolored subungual detritus. Treatment is conservative and consists of periodically trimming the nail carefully, although in more refractory cases, excision of the nail and matrix may be necessary. Koilonychia, or spoon-shaped nails, occurs in cases of iron deficiency anemia. Onychorrhexis consists of marked longitudinal striations in the nail and is often associated with nutritional disorders or rheumatoid arthritis.

Finally, trauma to the nail matrix can lead to a number of deformities (e.g., splits, ridges, pits), although they are usually asymptomatic.

MISCELLANEOUS SUBUNGUAL/ PARAUNGUAL LESIONS

Osteoid Osteoma

A benign bone lesion, common in children and young adults, osteoid osteoma produces recurrent pain attacks that are usually relieved by aspirin. Focal tenderness results from pressure on the involved nail plate, but due to the paucity of symptoms, the lesion is frequently not diagnosed. X-rays are usually diagnostic and show a central round radiopaque nidus surrounded by a thin, rarefied zone. Treatment consists of surgical excision under local anesthesia. Consultation is recommended. Subungual osteomas, also an uncommon tumor seen mostly in children and young adults, produces few long-term symptoms other than separation and deformity of the nail. X-rays are confirmatory, and the treatment of choice is surgical excision under local anesthesia with preservation of the nail, if possible.

A number of rare lesions may also be visible through the nail plate. For instance, a small, round bluish-red lesion that is paroxysmally painful, especially on exposure to cold, suggests a subungual glomus. Treatment consists of surgical removal of the distal nail plate and curettage of the tumor. Warts may also be located subungually and in this position can erode the adjacent tuft. Treatment is surgical excision. A subungual abscess may first be noted by the presence of a small whitish area underneath the nail bed, which represents the pus collection. Decompression by removal of the overlying nail or perforation with a dental drill or 18-gauge needle is curative. Rarely, a melanoma may be present as a discolored nail bed and should prompt a biopsy.

Periungual lesions include fibromas, warts, corns, and granuloma pyogenicum. The three former conditions are discussed in Chapter 4. A granuloma pyogenicum consists of an exuberant mass of granulation tissue overlying an ingrown toenail. Treatment is excisional biopsy of the pseudotumor and removal of the nail edge and its underlying matrix.

Paronychia

The distal phalanx of the toe may become inflamed or infected. The nail or bone itself may be involved. Etiologies include trauma, diabetes, and immunosuppression. Fungal and bacterial agents may also be involved.

Treatment consists of incision and drainage followed by povidone-iodine soaks four times a day. A topical antibiotic preparation can also be applied. Systemic antibiotics should be reserved for cellulitis extending to the metatarsophalangeal joint.

PIGMENTATION CHANGES

Toenails, like fingernails, are affected by systemic disease. A blue or azure lunula occurs in argyria. Diffuse melanosis suggests Addison's disease, neoplasia, hemochromatosis, or the adverse effects of chemotherapy (using quinacrine, antimalarials, etc.). Single or multiple white lines across the nail (Mees' lines) are found in arsenic and other heavy metal poisoning. White discoloration (leukonychia) has many causes, including autosomal dominant inheritance; hypoalbuminemia (Muehrcke's lines) is one well-known acquired cause. Others include trauma, cirrhosis, rheumatoid arthritis, and diabetes. A sudden interruption in matrix vascularity as a result of myocardial disease produces one or more white lines across the nail (Beau's lines). Gray discoloration occurs with chronic mercury poisoning. Yellow nails are associated with lymphatic edema from neoplasia or hypoplasia. Blackish discoloration of a nail may represent a melanotic whitlow or subungual hematoma if trauma has occurred. Half-and-half nails (Lindsay nails) are characterized by a deep reddish distal color and a white proximal portion. They are seen in patients with renal or liver failure. Terry's nails (deep red distal one-quarter and white proximal three-quarters) are seen in chronic liver disorders or connective tissue disorders.

BIBLIOGRAPHY

1. Yale JR: Yale's Podiatric Medicine, 3rd ed. Baltimore, Williams & Wilkins, 1987, pp 131–246.

Chapter 6

HALLUX

Richard B. Birrer, M.D.

HALLUX ABDUCTO VALGUS

This term denotes lateral (fibular) deviation of the great toe in association with prominence of the medial portion of the first metatarsal head, which tends to be a constant feature (Fig. 1). The complex deformity of hallux valgus needs to be distinguished from a bunion, which refers to the acute swelling or chronic tumefaction of the bursa overlying the first metatarsophalangeal joint. A bunion may or may not accompany hallux valgus. Though the condition may be associated in 30% of cases with a number of inherited problems such as hypermobile joints, Ehlers-Danlos disease, splaying of the forefoot, or metatarsus primus varus, it is almost exclusively a consequence of either short, narrow shoes with pointed toes and high heels or tight-fitting stockings or socks. The complex is far more common in females than males for the former reason, although some studies suggest a genetic predilection for the disorder. Over time, there are accommodative changes seen in the cartilage, articular ligaments, sesamoids, tendons, and joint capsule that form the first metatarsophalangeal joint. Normally both feet are affected, although usually one side has a more marked degree of deformity and symptoms.

The pathogenesis of hallux valgus consists of gradual lateral inclination of the great toe, pushing on the second, third, and fourth toes so that there is gradual fibular drift of these toes. The first, second, and third metatarsals tend to adduct; the fourth and fifth abduct. Atrophy of the exposed condylar cartilage of the metatarsal and phalanx is present. The sesamoids are displaced laterally into the first intermetatarsal space. This migration causes the sesamoids to undergo chondromalacia as well as to erode the cristae under the first metatarsal head, leading to denudation and ulceration. There is valgus rotation of the phalanx as it slips over or under its immediate fibular fellow. Subluxation of the first metatarsophalangeal joint causes the great toe to slide toward the axis of the foot and the metatarsal head to slip toward the mid axis of the body. Usually less than 50% of the metatarsal will articulate with its proximal phalanx. The soft tissues of the great toe undergo progressive accommodative shortening and lengthening of the lateral and medial sides, respectively. With degeneration of the joint's cartilaginous surface as well as recurrent microtrauma due to abnormal joint biomechanics, greater surface incongruity occurs, and exostosis, osteophytes, and early degenerative joint disease develop.

Shoe friction and irritative tension of the medial collateral ligament of the first metatarsophalangeal joint lead to chronic inflammation of the overlying bursa and further proliferation of fibrotic and osteoblastic activity. Once the resistance of normal bone structure and function has been partially removed, the unbalanced pulls of the flexor, extensor, adductor, and abductor hallucis muscles complete the process through their unopposed contractions. It is not uncommon to see the great toe in marked lateral deviation, held in extension away from the ground due to the bowstring effect of the extensor hallucis longus.

The symptoms of hallux valgus are related not necessarily to the degree of deformity but rather to complications. Repeated pressure and irritation from constricting shoe wear usually

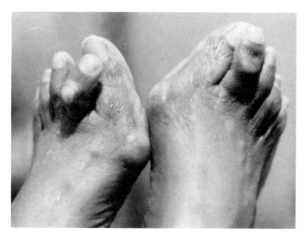

FIGURE 1. Bilateral hallux valgus with overlap of the second toe.

lead to pain and inflammation. Pressure over the sensory nerves may occasionally cause paresthesias on the medial aspect of the toe. In time, there is development of bunions, corns, calluses, septic bursitis, and occasionally septic arthritis due to the occurrence of a sinus or fistula tract. There is pain typically in the region of the sesamoids secondary to lateral displacement and degenerative changes.

Radiographs taken when the patient is weight bearing are confirmatory when the intermetatarsal angle is greater than 8 degrees and the metatarsophalangeal angle is greater than 15 degrees. The head of the first metatarsal is usually irregular, flat, and broad, and osteophytic spurs may be seen at the joint margins. There may be trabecular hypertrophy, joint effusion, and an irregular, dense, subarticular sclerotic line under the base of the proximal phalanx. Soft tissue swelling may overlie the deformed joint, which may represent bursal inflammation. Occasionally degeneration and calcification along the medial aspect are noted. The sesamoids will be displaced, and degenerative changes such as spurs and osteophytes occur. The differential diagnosis should include forms of arthritis such as rheumatoid, gout, and gonorrhea.

Therapeutic management of hallux valgus depends on the symptomatology, degree of deformity, extent of pathology, and presence of complicating factors. The majority of mild to moderate cases can be conservatively treated with good results. A bunion shield can be fashioned from tube foam, latex, or adhesive felt in such a manner that the pressure forces on the medial aspect of the first metatarsophalangeal joint are displaced circumferentially to noninvolved areas (Fig. 2). If adhesive felt is used, it is important to bevel the edge so that transition from felt to normal skin tissue is smooth and does not provide a focus for further hyperkeratotic reaction. Anti-inflammatory agents (e.g., aspirin) are also useful during the acute phase. Overlying hyperkeratotic tissue should be carefully pared down with a No. 15 scalpel blade. If there is a high degree of suspicion of an underlying bursitis, injection of a long-acting steroid (e.g., methylprednisolone acetate) is acceptable. A night splint and spaces between the first and second toe should also be prescribed, as should regular active and passive rehabilitative exercises perhaps in conjunction with low-voltage stimulation. Finally, the patient's footwear should be carefully examined and modified when appropriate: the toe box and shoe width should be adequate, the heel low, and socks and stockings loose. Shoes should be leather so that they can be modified by stretching to relieve pressure points. Without these latter changes, the therapeutic regimen will fail.

Surgical therapy is reserved for those who have severely symptomatic deformities and who

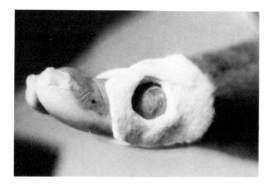

FIGURE 2. Adhesive felt bunion shield for hallux valgus.

have failed an adequate trial of conservative management (i.e., 6–12 months). Because there are over 100 surgical operations for hallux valgus and its attendant complications, this choice should be handled in association with a specialist. Preferred techniques include the Silver, Chevron, McBride, Akin, Lapidus, Mc-Keever, Mitchell, Keller, Akin, Mayo-Stone, and Hoffman procedures. Surgical complications are not infrequent: metatarsalgia, floppy great toe, stress fracture of the lesser metatarsal rays, recurrence, development of hallux varus, adhesive neuritis and tendinitis, infection, dehiscence, and hemorrhage can occur. Once again, rational footwear must be presented postoperatively in order to minimize recurrence.

HALLUX RIGIDUS

Limited range of motion of the first metatarsophalangeal joint due to previous trauma has been variously termed hallux regularis, hallux limitus, hallux flexis, hallux nonextensus, metatarsus primus elevatus, and dorsal bunion. In addition to trauma, other etiologies consist of rheumatoid arthritis, gout, hallux valgus, and hereditary factors. The condition is usually unilateral and more common in young adult males than females. There may be a single episode of severe trauma (e.g., stubbing of toe, kicking a hard object, or falling from a height), although more commonly, recurrent microtrauma is at fault (e.g., low-cut shoes with a tight toe box). Predisposing factors include a long, dorsally tilted first metatarsal ray, pes valgus planus, a forward projection big toe, and obesity. The patient usually complains of pain around the joint, especially upon tiptoeing or during the push-off phase of ambulation. The physical examination notes painful limitation, particularly of extension and flexion. Pain and tenderness are usually located dorsolaterally and may be associated with small amounts of erythema and edema. The patient may walk with an abducted gait or with the distal phalanx dorsiflexed, which serves as an accommodative fulcrum during gait.

Pathologically there is periarticular fibrosis with associated changes of ligaments and tendons as well as accommodative muscular spasms. Radiographically there are narrowing of the metatarsophalangeal joint space and development of spurs, lipping, and osteophytes at the articular margins, particularly the dorsal aspect of the first metatarsal head. The family doctor may also discover either a thickened hallucis longus tendon as it crosses the dorsal spur of the first metatarsal head or a fluctulant swelling on the plantar aspect of the joint, which is most likely a subcutaneous adventitial cyst secondary to constant friction. In rare cases, there may be complete ankylosis of the articulation. The differential diagnosis should include gout and rheumatoid arthritis.

The injection of 1–2 ml of anesthetic (e.g., lidocaine, bupivacaine hydrochloride) and 0.25–0.5 ml long-acting steroid (e.g., methylprednisolone acetate) results in immediate pain relief, relaxation of periarticular tissues, and long-term improvement of joint function. Traction with some basic range-of-motion exercises should also be started. A foot appliance can be fashioned from rigid metal or an acrylic polymer with the ultimate goal of shifting the weight to the lateral aspect of the foot. A Thomas or Denver heel, Jones bar, rigid shank, and extended counter will accomplish the same goals. Complete splinting of the joint through the use of a steel insole or an inlay appliance with a longitudinal portion extending just behind the sesamoids is also quite effective. Surgical intervention is reserved for a joint with no function or for cases of failed conservative therapy (see Chapter 20).

BIBLIOGRAPHY

1. Coughlin MJ: Etiology and treatment of the bunionette deformity. AAOS Instr Course Lect 39:37–48, 1990.
2. Evanski PM, Reinherz RP: Easing the pain of common foot problems. Patient Care 25:38–53, 1991.
3. Hawkins BJ, Haddad RJ: Hallux rigidus. Clin Sports Med 7:37–50, 1988.
4. Mann RA: The great toe. Orthop Clin North Am 20:519–534, 1989.
5. Silferskjöld JP: Common foot problems. Postgrad Med 89:183–188, 1991.

Chapter 7

SMALL TOES

Richard B. Birrer, M.D.

CORNS

The dorsal aspect of the smaller toes at the proximal and distal interphalangeal level and the lateral border of the fifth toe are common sites for hard corns. Corns can also occur on the terminal ends of the toes, especially if there is an associated flexion or mallet toe deformity. Corns may occur at other areas due to frictional irritation of the shoe against a phalangeal condyle, bony prominence, unreduced dislocation, or exostosis. Differences in toe length (e.g., fifth toe) may also be responsible for the formation of soft corns in the interdigital web spaces secondary to the pressure of a proximal phalangeal base and the head of a metatarsal against a condyle of a contiguous toe or vice versa. The diagnosis and treatment of corns are detailed elsewhere (see Chapters 4 and 20).

MALLET TOE DEFORMITY

Contracture of the distal interphalangeal toe joint in plantar flexion has been termed a mallet toe (Fig. 1). The deformity may be fixed or dynamically flexible and is usually limited to lesser digits of the foot (i.e., the second, third, or fourth), although the condition may be bilateral. High-heeled, pointed-toe shoes aggravate the deformity. The clinical exam reveals proximal interphalangeal joint flexion and one or more complications such as nail deformity or end corn or dorsal corn formation. The latter conditions are due to abnormal frictional irritation against the shoe or walking surface.

Treatment of mallet toe may be conservative or surgical. At a minimum, the shoe should

be roomy and well fitted, with a high, wide toe box and crepe soles in order to avoid pressure on the toes. A metatarsal bar or an insole (Plastazote) may be added to distribute pressure on the plantar aspect of the foot. Protective pads from moleskin, adhesive, or felt foam can be custom designed to protect the distal tuft or the dorsal aspect of the toe. An elastic sling can be made from similar materials and used to reduce the flexion deformity. A program of daily manipulation and stretching of the toes by the patient will help flexibility and delay a fixed deformity. A specialist should be consulted for surgical correction (e.g., flexor tenotomy, fusion, arthrotomy) of a fixed deformity.

HAMMER TOE (DIGITUS FLEXUS) DEFORMITY

Hyperextension of the distal interphalangeal joint in combination with a rigid flexion deformity of the proximal interphalangeal defines this deformity. Malposition of the proximal phalanx on the metatarsal head and contraction of the metatarsophalangeal capsule in dorsiflexion (claw toe) are commonly associated. Hammer toes may be fixed or flexible. The second toe is often involved because it is the longest toe and therefore easily traumatized by short or extremely pointed shoes or short stockings. The condition is often associated with hallux abducto valgus, rheumatoid arthritis and osteoarthritis. Complications include the development of corns, calluses, and bursitis over the proximal interphalangeal joint. Claw toes may also be fixed or flexible and are often complicated by the

45

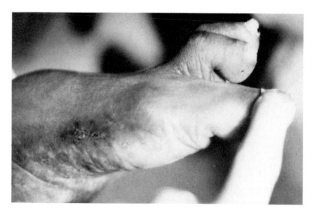

FIGURE 1. Mallet toes.

development of corns on the dorsum over the proximal interphalangeal joint or at the tuft of the involved toe.

Hammer toes may be either congenital or acquired, the latter being associated primarily with abnormal biomechanics. A short first metatarsal ray, as seen in a cavus foot, results in the increased transfer of weight to the second toe, with eventual formation of the deformity. In addition, in cavus foot there is decreased motor strength of the extensor digitorum brevis that causes weakening of normal extensor power and encouragement of hammer toe formation. Finally, neurologic conditions that weaken the anterior tibialis muscle and lead to extensor substitution (e.g., poliomyelitis) may also produce the classic hammer-toe posture. In time, contracture of the flexor and extensor tendons, fasciae, and collateral ligaments develops, and the skin of the plantar surface becomes contracted and very often fissured. The joints become enlarged, deformed, and occasionally ankylosed. X-ray examination may reveal calcification of the overlying bursa or a calcified sinus tract. There may be sequestration and local bone necrosis. Finally, osteophytic spurring and lipping may be seen.

The successful management of hammer toe may be either conservative or surgical, depending on the degree of deformity, the number of joints involved, whether the deformity is fixed or flexible, the presence of complications, and the age and health of the patient. Palliative treatment consists of custom fitting the appropriate adhesive felt, foam rubber, or similar device to protect pressure areas from development of hyperkeratosis. Forced extension of the toes can be ensured by the fitting of a toe crest pad on the plantar surface (Fig. 2). A plantar splint with a dorsal elastic sling may also be used for considerable improvement. Finally, it is important that the patient's footwear be carefully examined and an extra-depth toe box be prescribed. Inlaid-depth shoes may also allow sufficient freedom and relief of pressure in the forefoot. Moldable plastic materials and silicone products can be used along with tube gauze to produce an accommodative appliance for the palliative management of hammer toes (e.g., Budin splints and the double-ring hammer-toe device of Polokoff).

A number of surgical techniques can correct hammer toes and claw toes; these approaches should be handled by consultation. Examples include proximal hemiphalangectomy (DuVries and Mann method), Kelikian syndactylation, distal hemiphalangectomy, forced straightening, metatarsal head resection,

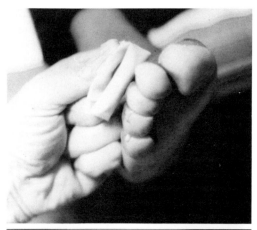

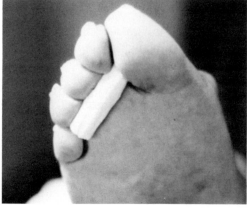

FIGURE 2. Toe crest pads.

diaphysectomy or waist resection of the proximal phalanx, and osteotomy (Tierny's method) (see Chapter 20).

TRIGGER TOES

Tenosynovitis of the flexor hallucis longus tendon with resultant triggering due to rupture of its central fibers has been noted in ballet dancers and joggers. The athlete will usually complain of tenderness, perhaps swelling, and painful clicking, snapping, or popping during the exacerbating activity. Careful, controlled injection of a long-acting steroid may be useful (see Chapter 20), although surgical lysis of adhesions and the removal of the entrapment are often necessary.

UNDERLAPPING TOES (CURLED UNDERTOES)

This deformity needs to be distinguished from mallet toes and claw toes. Overriding and underriding toes are usually acquired and frequently associated with the development of a hallux abducto valgus deformity (Fig. 3). If the hallux underrides the second toe, there are usually atrophy and discoloration of the toe nail due to the prolonged forces of weight bearing. Overriding of the second toe by the hallux causes severe contraction of the adductor hallucis, joint capsule, and articular ligaments. The third, fourth, and fifth toes may also overlap or underride, particularly if there is hypermobility of the foot. Most of the deformities occur at the interphalangeal joint with abnormal metatarsophalangeal joints. The third and fourth toes tend to underlap both one another and the second toe, whereas the fifth toe often overlaps the fourth, although underlapping is not uncommon. In addition, there are associated contracture of the skin, joint capsule, and extensor tendon. Complications include the development of soft and hard corns and dystrophic changes of nails due to repeated trauma. Treatment depends on the degree and type of deformity, age, and overall health status of the patient. For instance, overlapping of the second toe due to hallux abducto valgus usually requires treatment of the hallux in order for the second toe to resume its neutral position. Regardless of severity, if the deformity is flexible, a trial of conservative therapy is still warranted.

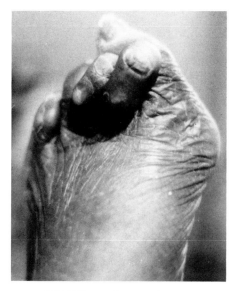

FIGURE 3. Overlapping toes.

Adequacy of footwear, particularly a sufficient toe box, is paramount, and the use of tailored splints, removable crests, or similar appliances located on functional insoles will go far in improving the condition (e.g., transverse Budin splint). Surgery should be reserved for the most refractory cases and be handled in consultation. Examples include metatarsal head resection, diaphysectomy, hemiphalangectomy of the proximal portion of the proximal phalanx, tenectomy, tenotomy, capsulotomy, syndactyly, arthroplasty, or a variety of combinations of these methods.

PARAUNGUAL LESIONS

The most common paraungual lesions of the small toes are nail groove corns. Gentle curetting with a curette of 1–2 mm is usually sufficient, although lesions associated with the fibular side of the fifth toe may be more troublesome. The lesion is usually due to frictional shoe pressure secondary to tight-fitting shoe gear that squares off the toes. Gentle periodic paring and use of liberal open-toed shoe or one with a deeper toe box are mostly curative, although removal of the entire nail and matrix (Syme procedure) may be required. The most common subungual lesion is an end corn adjacent to the free nail edge due to a complicating, fixed hammer toe deformity. Correction of the hammer toe is usually all that is required.

MISCELLANEOUS CONDITIONS

Repetitive microtrauma, common among long-distance runners and joggers, may be seen in the small toes as an asymptomatic subungual brownish-black lesion due to micro-hemorrhage (see Chapter 13). The condition has been termed runner's toe. The differential diagnosis must include malignant melanoma and pigment-producing fungal and bacterial infections. Ulcerations between toe web spaces of the small toes and the tips of the toes should suggest peripheral neuropathy or a microvascular impairment.

The small toes are the most frequently involved in rheumatoid arthritis and less frequently in gout and arthritis. There may be an associated interphalangeal joint flexion contracture or fixation in extension. The initial presentation of psoriasis and rheumatoid arthritis may involve the isolated swelling of the small toe in the form of linear periostitis. A relatively rare condition seen primarily in blacks is the spontaneous autoamputation of the small toes, termed ainhum. The fourth and fifth toes are most commonly involved, though the second and third ones can be affected, as can the fingers. Over a period of several years, a narrow, bandlike constriction develops, usually at the base of the fourth or fifth toe, which starts medially and spreads progressively plantarward and dorsolaterally. The condition may be bilateral; it affects both men and women in their mid-40s and tends to be symptomless. Treatment is expectant.

BIBLIOGRAPHY

1. Coughlin MJ: Subluxation and dislocation of the second metatarsophalangeal joint. Orthop Clin North Am 20: 535–551, 1989.
2. Coughlin MJ: Lesser toe abnormalities. In Chapman M (ed): Operative Orthopedics. Philadelphia, J.B. Lippincott, 1989, pp 1765–1776.
3. Evanski PM, Reinherz RP: Easing the pain of common foot problems. Patient Care 25:38–53, 1991.
4. Mann RA: Pathological anatomy of claw and hammer toes. J Bone Joint Surg 72A:305, 1990.
5. Richardson EG: The foot in adolescents and adults. In Crenshaw AH (ed): Campbell's Operative Orthopaedics, 7th ed. St. Louis, Mosby-Year Book, 1987, pp 937–948.

Chapter 8

METATARSALS

Richard B. Birrer, M.D.

ANATOMY

The many anatomic relations among the metatarsals are important for understanding pertinent pathophysiology. Even though the fifth metatarsal is usually the longest in the foot, the most important relationship exists between the first and second. Twenty-five to 30% of individuals have an "index plus/minus" type of foot in which the first and second metatarsals are approximately equal in length, whereas the forward ends of the other three metatarsals progressively diminish in length. Fifty-five to 60% of people exhibit the "index minus" prototype in which the first metatarsal is shorter than the second. Finally, in the "index plus" conformation, the first metatarsal is longer, and the forward ends of the others decrease progressively.

PHYSIOLOGY

Under normal physiologic conditions, the heads of all metatarsals should rest evenly on the floor in the standing position regardless of the type of forefoot, particularly in the tiptoe position. In one study of 100 normal people, the use of a podoscope demonstrated that 30% use all metatarsals, 28.5% the first three metatarsals, 28.5% the lateral metatarsals, and 13% the central rays. These static findings are preserved during the dynamic aspects of gait, and it is the biomechanical alteration of the metatarsal area that is the most frequent cause of pain in the forefoot (e.g., metatarsalgia). The pathomechanics of metatarsal pain can be classified according to anatomic location and the distribution of weight on the metatarsal supports, diffuse or focal. Diffuse overload occurs in anterior support problems; focal overload follows first-ray overload and insufficiency syndrome, and central ray overload and insufficiency syndrome.

METATARSALGIA

Anterior support overload occurs in the equinus foot, the cavus foot, and the foot in a high-heeled shoe. Eighty-five to 90% of metatarsalgia occurs in females. Shoes with elevated heels greatly increase the force exerted against the metatarsal heads. In addition, a cramped, pointed toe box crowds the toes together in dorsiflexion so that the metatarsal condyles lose normal anterior support from the toes. These changes can be readily demonstrated with a Harris foot mat. The success of all therapy in this situation depends on wearing a low-heeled shoe with an adequate toe box.

Equinus foot deformity caused by contracture of the Achilles tendon from congenital as well as inherited disorders (e.g., cerebrovascular accidents, poliomyelitis) results in limited dorsiflexion and consequent overload of the anterior support on the metatarsal heads. Abnormal increases of the plantar arch in the form of a cavus foot result in the maldistribution of weight at the heel as well as at the metatarsal heads. The associated subluxation and sometimes dislocation of the toes also aggravate metatarsalgia by removing normal toe support of the metatarsals. Finally, in equinus, the metatarsal heads are generally the first point of contact with the floor, again increasing the symptoms of metatarsalgia. Because gait malfunction (i.e., dynamic cavus

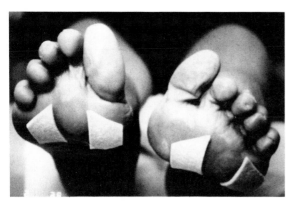

FIGURE 1. Metatarsal pontoons made of adhesive felt.

foot) appears before pathologic manifestation (i.e., structured cavus foot), early diagnosis and treatment can prevent many of the principal biomechanic disturbances caused by the deformity. The differential diagnosis should also include systemic causes such as gout and rheumatoid arthritis (i.e., degenerative, rheumatoid, psoriatic).

Treatment

The therapeutic approach to anterior support overload may be either conservative or surgical. If there is no underlying foot deformity, the recommendation is to prepare a metatarsal bar or pontoon fashioned out of adhesive felt or foam rubber (Fig. 1). The device is placed behind or adjacent to the metatarsal heads in order to diffuse frictional pressure. A low-heeled shoe and stretching of the calcaneus are imperative in order to reduce frictional irritation. In the child with a dynamic cavus foot, normal gait through regular rehabilitative exercises must be established, particularly walking barefoot on a smooth floor. The emphasis here is to impact the floor with the heel rather than the ball of the foot. Supplementary arch supports as well as a metatarsal bar and pontoon are useful. Physical therapy can be supplemented by diathermy, ultrasound, hydrotherapy, and massage in order to minimize fibrotic contraction (see Chapter 20). Once there is structural deformity present in the soft tissue or bones, consultation with a qualified specialist should be sought in order to determine the appropriate course. Examples of soft tissue operations include the method of Steindler and Camera; operations for skeletal deformities consist of arthrodesis and the metatarsectomy method of Lelievre.

FIRST-RAY OVERLOAD

Overload of the first ray occurs under two circumstances. The first involves a very long big toe that is joined to a strong metatarsal. With repetitive microtrauma to the metatarsophalangeal joint, enhanced by an insufficient toe box and metatarsus elevatus, osteoarthritis of the joint develops, leading to hallux rigidus. The second pathogenetic mechanism of first-ray overload involves frontal load imbalance of the head of the metatarsal and the sesamoids. Acute overload can follow a fall on the tiptoes or the sudden application of brake pressure, as in a traffic accident. Repetitive microtrauma resulting from dancing, particularly ballet, can lead to front load imbalance. A chronic syndrome can result when the angle that the first metatarsal forms with the floor is greater than 25 degrees. The most common causes are high heels and the presence of a cavus foot.

The patient usually complains of chronic pain, particularly a dull ache. The clinical exam discloses pain at the level of the head of the first metatarsal; the practitioner may also note some indurated edema and limitation of motion. The internal arch is usually increased, the condyles of the first metatarsals are prominent, and the big toe is held in hyperextension. Hyperkeratosis, in the form of tylomata and helomata, is characteristic in the region of the overload zone. In more advanced cases, the bursitis may be noted by crepitus, a small ulcer, or the sinus tract. Radiographs usually reveal hypertrophy of the margins of the first metatarsophalangeal joint, narrowing of the joint space, and lipping, exostosis, and osteophytic spurs of the articular surfaces. Soft tissue swelling is usually noted in longer-term cases, and the bursa may be fibrotic and calcified.

Treatment

Palliative treatment consists of either custom fitting an orthotic, pontoon, or cushion in the form of a half-moon that protects the overload zone or designing an insole that has a retrocapital support. Diathermy can be applied in selected cases; especially with complicating bursitis, a long-acting steroid-anesthetic combination can be beneficial (see Chapter 20).

Anti-inflammatory agents are useful supplements. If the underlying etiology is repetitive microtrauma, then well-fitted, firm-soled footwear with an anterior heel or Jones bar is helpful. Surgery should be reserved for the most refractory cases after several months of conservative therapy. Standard surgical interventions include the Jones operation, metatarsal base osteotomy, and sesamoidectomy.

FIRST-RAY INSUFFICIENCY

Insufficiency of the first ray causes dysfunction of the foot with overloading of the other rays, particularly of the second and third metatarsals, a condition variously described as "open foot," splayfoot, metatarsus varus, transverse or anterior flatfoot, and Morton's syndrome. Acutely, such static alterations result in march fractures or Deutschlander's disease. Long-term effects seen in this syndrome result in overlapping of the toes. The causes of first-ray insufficiency are congenital (e.g., posterior placement of the sesamoids, a shortened first metatarsal, or varus deviation of the first metatarsal), soft tissue dysfunction (e.g., laxity of the Lisfranc ligament), dislocation of the sesamoids, flattening of the longitudinal arch, and such iatrogenic causes as Hueter-Mayo operation (i.e., removing and remodeling the metatarsal head), metatarsal osteotomy (which usually shortens the first ray), and a variety of operations that diminish the strength of the big toe (e.g., Brandes-Keller operation). Regardless of etiology, insufficiency of the first ray must be borne by the adjacent rays.

Acutely, the insufficiency is manifested by sudden decompensation in the form of a march fracture. There is a sudden onset of intense pain in the second or third metatarsal due to a spontaneous fracture associated with long periods of walking or as a consequence of the marching that is typical of military personnel. The afflicted individual must often stop walking, and swelling may occur over the dorsal aspect of the affected foot. The condition is unilateral and most commonly affects the second ray, though the third and fourth may be involved as well. Radiologically, except for an obviously shortened ray, there are usually no acute changes noted, although 2–3 weeks after the injury, a periosteal reaction occurs around a clear line at the union of the distal and middle thirds of the bone.

Deutschlander, who originally described the condition in 1921, noted three phases: the acute phase, which lasts 2 months and is characterized by pain and usually negative radiographs; a periosteal reaction lasting about 3 months, during which time the radiographs are positive; and a reparative, or healing, phase of approximately 4 months in which the bone structure returns to normal. The availability of bone scan techniques makes the earlier diagnosis of march fracture possible even within the first week.

Progressive first-ray insufficiency causes characteristic pathophysiologic changes. A thick diffuse callus or hyperkeratotic area develops under the heads of the second, third, and fourth metatarsals in over 75% of patients. The hyperkeratosis is often associated with submetatarsal bursitis. Thickening of the cortex of the second metatarsal may also be seen radiographically, along with stress fractures. Finally, the abnormal biomechanics can cause dorsal dislocation and subluxation of the second and third toes, resulting in claw deformity.

Treatment

Treatment of first-ray insufficiency depends on etiology as well as degree of deformity. In the acute form, treatment of a lesser metatarsal stress fracture is best managed by application of a posterior splint or soft case (e.g., Unna boot) or a surgical adhesive strapping in combination with rest, elevation, ice, and anti-inflammatory agents. The cast should remain in place for two to three weeks; thereafter, progressive ambulation with taping or a shoe with a rigid sole and supportive inlay is advised. Once healing has occurred, attention must then be directed to the underlying etiology in order to prevent recurrence.

Treatment for the chronic form may be palliative or surgical. Analgesics and anti-inflammatories should be incorporated during the initial visit in order to relieve intense pain and discomfort. The hyperkeratotic area should be carefully trimmed and a suitable orthosis fashioned to balance the variation and provide support to the forefoot. The use of an elastic metatarsal bandage of 3–5 cm in width around the metatarsals in an attempt to reduce their distal divergence and to correct the varus of the first metatarsal or the valgus deformity of the fifth is not useful. A number of orthotics can be custom fitted, including a metatarsal bar or anterior heel (i.e., an elevated transverse bar of the shoe sole situated behind the central metatarsal heads) that diffuses the excess pressure causing the metatarsalgia. A Morton's device consists of an insole that has a prolongation beneath the first metatarsal of the big toe in order to correct the insufficient first ray. The Martorell arch support consists of not only a metatarsal bar but also a toe crest placed in the digital plantar fold in order to prevent foot slippage on the insole surface and to provide further pressure dissipation from the metatarsal heads. These supports may also be supplemented by dorsal digital splints that force plantar toe flexion. Such adhesive felts or sponge rings are placed at the base of the toes so that, with normal pressure, the toe is forced downward.

These therapeutic modalities should be supplemented by an active physiotherapy program for the best functional result, regardless of whether there is surgical intervention or not. It is essential to develop the flexor muscles of the forefoot, since a great tendency exists in this syndrome to produce toe dorsiflexion. The exercise program consists of both active and passive components. Active exercises should be performed in a tub of warm water and should begin with a full range of motion emphasizing plantar flexion. In particular, the exercises can be done on a small wooden platform placed inside the tub so that the metatarsal heads rest on the edge of the platform and the toes overhang. Thereafter, a number of mechanical exercises are routinely practiced for eight repetitions. Examples are towel grasps, pencil curls, and small ball pick-ups. An exercise session should include a short period of barefoot ambulation on a smooth surface. During the push-off phase, all the toes must make surface contact, especially the big toe. A surface of wet sand is extremely valuable, as it clearly demarcates the contact points of the five toes and reinforces the importance of plantar flexion. Passive exercises include manipulation and postural modifications. The ball of the foot and the metatarsophalangeal articulations of each toe should be gently, but progressively, squeezed systematically in order to overcome the stiffness and inflammation of metatarsal areas and the dorsal retractions of musculotendinous units in the region. Postural treatments include either bending the foot in strong plantar flexion when the patient is seated or adopting a knee attitude and producing the same plantar flexion.

A good 6-month trial of such conservative treatment should be applied rigorously before surgical consultation is sought. Discussion of the surgical management of first-ray insufficiency syndrome is beyond the scope of this work, although, in general, the approach depends on the type of deformity and its attendant complications. Thus, depending on circumstances, the first metatarsal may be lengthened, realigned, or fused, or the remaining metatarsals shortened by resection or osteotomy.

CENTRAL-RAY OVERLOAD

Central-ray overload syndrome rarely involves a single metatarsal ray but rather affects several, in diminishing order from the second to the fourth metatarsals. The syndrome is typically seen in compensatory combination with insufficiency of the first ray. Single, central-ray metatarsal overloads occur congenitally or when there is loss of proximal articulation dorsiflexion—a condition most commonly seen in the fourth ray. The patient usually complains of pain in the area of the inflamed condyle. Clinical examination reveals the appearance of hyperkeratosis in the form of corns and calluses. In the chronic situation, there may be a bursitis that can become infected and progression to an ulceration, if not treated early. Treatment for central-ray overload syndrome is similar to that for first-ray insufficiency. Surgery should be reserved for failures of palliative modalities and usually involves osteotomy or condylectomy.

CENTRAL-RAY INSUFFICIENCY

Central-ray insufficiency syndrome is characterized by overload of the first and fifth metatarsals. The etiology may be congenital, neurologic, or iatrogenic. The most common congenital cause is aplasia of one or more metatarsal segments. The fourth metatarsal is usually involved with the deformity, becoming evident in early infancy or following cases of poliomyelitis. Clinically, the condition does not become symptomatic until later in childhood when the third and fifth toes deviate compensatorily, producing metatarsalgia. With few exceptions, the treatment of congenital insufficiency central-ray syndrome involves surgical removal of the entire ray and corresponding toe.

INTERDIGITAL NEUROMA

Interdigital plantar neuroma is a common cause of metatarsal pain with distinctive pathology. The condition has been variously referred to as Morton's disease, Morton's toe, Morton's metatarsalgia, and anterior metatarsalgia. It is frequently confused with first-metatarsal insufficiency syndrome. Classically, the condition affects adults 20–50 years of age, typically females (8:1 ratio), in the region of the fourth metatarsophalangeal articulation. Although most commonly unilateral, it may be bilateral. The patient complains of sharp, lancinating pain in the third and fourth metatarsal interspaces, with radiation of the pain toward the third and fourth toes. The pain may have a burning or electric shock sensation and occurs at rest, usually following a period of prolonged walking or strenuous foot exertion. The patient often attempts to relieve the discomfort by removing the shoes and massaging the feet. Initially the pain crises are intermittent, but over time they may become chronic in nature. The clinical exam tends to be unremarkable. Some pressure pain in the distal of the third and fourth interspaces may be noted when the soft parts are compressed. Compression of the adjacent bones may produce plantar pain. Rarely, a small tumor may be palpable in the affected area. Radiologic investigations are also unremarkable, because there are no fixed concomitant bony alterations. The differential diagnosis should include Deutschlander's disease (i.e., pain produced by pressure on the distal third-metatarsal diaphysis), Morton's syndrome, bursitis, tumors, stress fracture, and other causes of metatarsalgia (e.g., pain in the head of the involved metatarsal).

Pathogenetically, there is repetitive microtrauma to a branch of the lateral plantar nerve. Tight shoes, frequently noted in women, and certain professions such as ballet dancing are predisposing factors in the pathogenesis of the lesion. Strong evidence suggests that the particular branch of the lateral plantar nerve is congenitally enlarged, although other theories include neoplastic and vascular etiologies for the neuroma. The majority of cases of Morton's neuroma respond to conservative therapy. A rigid insole made preferably of metal, is carefully fitted to immobilize the metatarsals as well as compensate for any biomechanical dysfunction that may exist (e.g., flat feet or first-metatarsal insufficiency). Anti-inflammatory agents should also be prescribed. If the patient does not respond to this initial form of palliation, injection of anesthetic and corticosteroid (see Chapter 20) into the dorsal part of the foot at the point of pain is most beneficial. The treatment can be combined with short-wave diathermic applications. Several authors have also recommended large doses of vitamin B. For the refractory case, surgical extirpation of the pathologic area of the nerve is curative. Consultation with a specialist is advised.

SESAMOIDITIS

The first-metatarsal sesamoids may become inflamed spontaneously or from trauma. Physical examination reveals a trigger point beneath the metatarsal head that increases with dorsiflexion of the metatarsophalangeal joint. X-ray examination may show a fractured sesamoid and callus formation, but it must be remembered that, because sesamoids are frequently bipartite or tripartite, comparison films are recommended. Low-heeled shoes and a metatarsal bar proximal to the metatarsal head are usually satisfactory. In addition, conservative modalities include taping the great toe in slight plantar flex and prescribing nonsteroidal anti-inflammatory drugs. Surgical excision is reserved for chronic recurrent pain.

PERIARTHRITIS

Periarthritis between the first two metatarsophalangeal joints—also called the second-metatarsal interspace syndrome—manifests itself as a sharp pain in the distal second-metatarsal interspace. There may or may not be signs of local inflammation. The pain does not radiate; it worsens with ambulation, and it disappears at rest. Careful palpation reveals a trigger point in the second interspace that can be confirmed by the examiner's pinching the interspace. Injection of a combination of local anesthetic and long-acting steroid is not only diagnostic but also curative (see Chapter 20). Etiologically, there may be a short first ray; rarely will there be other changes. Intermittent forefoot dysfunction is the most common etiology and is usually secondary to poorly fitting or inappropriate footwear.

Symptoms of generalized synovitis in association with subluxation and dislocation of multiple metatarsophalangeal joints suggest a generalized disease process such as arthritis (see Chapter 15).

MISCELLANEOUS CAUSES
OF METATARSALGIA

A variety of neuropathic processes (e.g., cerebral palsy, poliomyelitis, Charcot-Marie-Tooth disease) increase the longitudinal and transverse arches of the foot so that the first and fifth metatarsals tend to lie more inferior in the horizontal plane than the central rays. Pathogenetically, there is an imbalance of the anterior tibial and peroneus longus muscles. Subcutaneous hygromata, hyperkeratotic zones, and incapacitating pain in the first and fifth metatarsals are characteristic, although chronically, trophic ulcers may develop in the same region. The underlying condition must be diagnosed and treated before manifestations in the feet can be addressed. Normally, palliative therapy in the form of orthotics produces beneficial results. Surgery should be reserved only for a failed trial of conservative therapy (of several months) and confirmation of a static lesion (e.g., nonprogressive).

BIBLIOGRAPHY

1. Brantingham JW, et al: Morton's neuroma. J Physiol Ther 14:317–322, 1991.
2. Evanski PM, Reinherz RP: Easing the pain of common foot problems. Patient Care 25:38–53, 1991.
3. Gould JS: Metatarsalgia. Orthop Clin North Am 20:553–562, 1989.
4. Scranton PE: Metatarsalgia: A clinical review of diagnosis and management. Foot Ankle 1:229, 1989.

Chapter 9

HEEL, SUBTALAR COMPLEX, AND ANKLE

Michael P. DellaCorte, D.P.M.,
and William F. Buffone, D.P.M.

HEEL

Plantar Fasciitis

Despite mythical connotations of vulnerability (i.e., Achilles heel), the heel of the foot has efficiently adapted to and successfully carried the human being through a long evolutionary process. The heel is not immune to injury, however, which usually presents as pain. Plantar pain may be due to plantar fasciitis or the formation and inflammation of calcaneal spurs. The process of spur formation has been termed heel spur syndrome. Repeated microtrauma of the plantar aponeurosis, occurring in a variety of running sports (e.g., football, soccer, jogging), especially in the unconditioned or obese individual, can cause straining of the posterior attachment and adjacent short muscles in the region of its posterior attachment to the medial tubercle on the plantar surface of the os calcis. The condition may be bilateral, although it is more commonly unilateral. Pain is more pronounced on initial weight bearing in the morning or after prolonged periods of sitting. At least 50% of these individuals have a calcaneal spur diagnosed on x-ray, although in only 25% will there, in actuality, be cause and effect. Clinical examination confirms diffuse tenderness in the region of the calcaneal tuberosity, particularly the medial side. Tenderness is usually not over the area of the spur.

Treatment is conservative. Aspirin or nonsteroidal anti-inflammatory drugs (NSAIDs) are useful in reducing the acute inflammation. Acutely, the lesion should be carefully strapped with surgical adhesive tape and tincture of benzoin (see Chapter 20). Thereafter, a custom-fitted medial arch support with heel dispersion is designed from adhesive, felt, foam, plastazote, or polypropylene so that the foot is held in inversion and adduction, thus reducing medial longitudinal arch stretch. A simple one-quarter-inch wedge may be effective, but in refractory cases, a carefully fitted transferable orthotic will be required. Injection therapy and physiotherapy may also help.

Heel Spur

Initially presenting as a periostitis, a calcaneal spur is an osseous extension of the medial process of the calcaneal tuberosity in a forward direction within the central plantar fascia. The etiology is presumed to be chronic traction of the plantar fascia and the flexor digitorum brevis, quadratus plantae, and abductor hallucis. Although the lesion may develop in a young athlete, the patient is usually an older obese adult in whom the plantar padding has thinned due to aging (see Chapter 11). The patient complains of an acutely painful heel, particularly on rising in the morning or following periods of rest (poststatic dyskinesia). Normally, the pain disappears after ambulation, only to reappear after prolonged amounts of walking and weight bearing.

The pain is described as the feeling of a nail or pin sticking in the foot, and is located at the medial tubercle on the plantar surface.

Palpation is helpful, including the stress maneuver of stretching the plantar fascia at its insertion site by dorsiflexing the digits at the metatarsophalangeal joints. Tenderness is pinpoint rather than diffuse, and the x-ray examination clearly demonstrates the spur formation emanating from the calcaneal tuberosity. Although not seen on conventional x-ray, the spur extends from medial to lateral, and absence of a spur suggests fasciitis. Spur size does not necessarily correlate with clinical findings. The differential diagnosis should include acute bursitis and plantar fasciitis, both of which may coexist with a spur. Gout and, rarely, bone tumors can also cause heel pain.

Treatment in the majority of cases is conservative and follows the guidelines outlined for the treatment of plantar fasciitis. In addition, a custom-fitted orthotic made from a suitable material can be used to displace pressure from the spur to the lateral zones. Injection of the trigger point should be reserved for the chronically recurrent situation but should be attempted before surgery (see Chapter 20). Surgical excision through a medial incision is indicated for refractory cases (minimum of 6 months' failed conservative therapy or intractable pain). Postoperatively, the patient is kept in a non-weight-bearing cast or splint for 3 weeks to prevent calcaneal fracture. Gradual weight bearing is then initiated in conjunction with postoperative biomechanical control of pronation with orthotics.

Heel Pain

Posterior heel pain can be due to calcaneal exostosis, retrocalcaneal bursitis, a short Achilles tendon, Achilles tendinitis, bursitis, and a variety of athletic injuries. Recurrent irritation and pressure to the posterior heel from poorly fitting shoes (e.g., sling-backs; high-heeled pumps; stiff, tight counters; athletic footwear typical of hockey and figure skating) constitute the most common etiology for the majority of these conditions, particularly in the young patient. In the older patient—most frequently females—chilblains, frostbite, and rheumatoid arthritis can lead to heel pain. With long-term, repeated injury there may be formation of visible "pump bumps," which represent the generic end state of a number of problems.

Athletic causes of posterior heel pain (jogger's heel) include strains of the Achilles tendon, fat pad atrophy, stress fracture, and

entrapment of the terminal branches of the posterior tibial nerve. Apophysitis of the calcaneus occurs in the pediatric age group.

Lateral heel pain is most frequently due to pathology involving the peroneal tendons, particularly subluxation or frank dislocation of the peroneus longus (see Chapter 13). Other causes include irregularities of the calcaneus and fibula, as well as static disorders.

Causes of **medial heel pain** include tarsal tunnel syndrome, strains of the tibialis posterior, and neurodynia of the medial calcaneal nerve. Compression of the posterior tibial nerve by the laciniate ligament can produce debilitating hyperesthesias along the medial plantar surface of the foot. Initially, there are both ill-defined discomfort and pain on the posterior aspect of the heel below the medial malleolus to the mid-tarsal zone. Over time, the pain becomes more severe, aching in quality, and aggravated by standing and weight bearing but also present at rest. Reproduction of the pain and discomfort during palpation in the region of the laciniate ligament, located about a finger's breadth below the medial malleolus, is highly suggestive. The disorder is confirmed by electromyographic studies of the nerve. Conservative treatment of the syndrome consists of custom-fitted orthotics, NSAIDs, and, if necessary, adhesive strapping. Such palliative therapy is usually sufficient in the initial stages of the syndrome. Chronically, surgical neurolysis may be necessary.

Retrocalcaneal Bursitis

Inflammation of the bursa lying between the Achilles tendon and the posterior border of the os calcis is termed retrocalcaneal bursitis, anterior Achilles bursitis, achillodynia, and Albert's disease. Trauma can cause acute bursitis; gout, rheumatoid arthritis, pes planus, and such infectious diseases as tuberculosis and gonorrhea can lead to chronic bursitis. Trauma usually occurs both directly and indirectly. A blow or kick to the heel is the most common direct cause; sudden jumps in gymnastics and running can indirectly strain the Achilles tendon. The clinical exam discloses localized tenderness at the sides of the tendon at its insertion site. The patient holds the foot in eversion to avoid dorsiflexion, and there may be some swelling and erythema evident at the tendon's lateral borders. Aspirin and NSAIDs are useful during the acute phase, as is a one-quarter-inch heel wedge. Heel immobilization by adhesive strapping is quite useful, and injection of a long-acting steroid and local anesthetic combination may be occasionally beneficial (see Chapter 20).

Achilles Bursitis

Inflammation of the posterior Achilles or precalcaneal bursa may also occur as a result of the predisposing factors already mentioned. The bursa, located between the skin and the Achilles tendon, may have bullae, fissures, and ulcerations associated with its chronic inflammation. The inflammation site is typically at the margin of the shoe counter, and chronic calcification may be noted on x-ray as will the formation of a calcaneal exostosis located at the attachment of the tendon. Over time, there may be enlargement of the posterior superior angle of the calcaneus, termed Haglund's deformity. This lesion, in turn, will aggravate the overlying bursitis. Pain is usually severe with any movement of the Achilles tendon, and, although the conservative modalities already mentioned for retrocalcaneal bursitis should be attempted, surgical removal of the exostosis is usually necessary.

Haglund's Deformity

Haglund's deformity is sometimes called "pump bump" because of its frequency among women who wear pump shoes. It is an osseous deformity of the posterior superior aspect of the calcaneus. The patient presents with pain over the osseous deformity. A subcutaneous bursa, a tyloma, or both may contribute to the patient's symptoms. Pain occurs on ambulation while wearing the offending shoe gear.

The etiology of the condition is pronation associated with several biomechanical problems (e.g., partially or fully compensated rearfoot varus, plantar-flexed first-ray insufficiency, or rigid forefoot valgus). As the calcaneus everts during stance phase, friction between the calcaneus and the shoe counter leads to the formation of the exostosis. Friction may also contribute to the formation of a corn or tyloma.

A prominence will be observed at the posterosuperior aspect of the calcaneus. There is pain upon palpation of the exostosis, tyloma, or bursa. X-ray examination reveals a prominent posterosuperior aspect of the calcaneus on the lateral view.

Treatment. Conservative treatment of Haglund's deformity can be achieved with padding, change of shoe gear, control of pronation with orthotics, and steroid injections (see Chapter 20).

If conservative treatment fails, surgical resection of the prominent posterosuperior aspect of the calcaneus is indicated. A linear incision is made over the prominence just lateral to the insertion of the Achilles tendon. Resection of the exostosis should be aggressive because of the high incidence of recurrence of the deformity. Postoperatively, the patient should be kept nonweightbearing for several weeks to guard against possible rupture of the Achilles tendon. The patient should also be placed in orthotics to decrease the incidence of recurrence.

Retrocalcaneal Exostosis and Tendocalcinosis of the Achilles Tendon

These two conditions can occur together or individually. The patient will complain of pain across the posterior aspect of the heel at the site of insertion of the Achilles tendon. The pain is described as a dull ache. A tender palpable exostosis and/or hypertrophied Achilles tendon may be present. One can usually elicit pain with range of motion. A lateral view x-ray of the heel is recommended on the initial visit. One may see either an exostosis emanating from the posterior central aspect of the calcaneus or calcifications within the Achilles tendon. Occasionally, the spur may fragment at the site of the insertion of the Achilles tendon. If these findings are not observed, a retrocalcaneal bursitis or a hypertrophied Achilles tendon may be the etiology of the symptoms.

Conservative treatment of these conditions may be achieved by padding, heel lifts, orthotics, and NSAIDs. Steroid injections are not recommended because of the proximity of insertion of the Achilles tendon. If all conservative treatment fails, surgical removal of the exostosis and/or removal of calcific deposits within the Achilles tendon may be required. A significant portion of the Achilles tendon insertion on the calcaneus may have to be detached in order to gain exposure to the retrocalcaneal exostosis. The exostosis can then be removed with an osteotome or power bur.

Postoperatively, the patient is kept four to five weeks nonweightbearing in an above-knee cast or splint, with the knee flexed and the foot in plantarflexion. Immobilization is required to allow for tenodesis of the Achilles tendon to the calcaneus.

For discussions of tibialis posterior strain and Achilles tendinitis, see Chapters 11 and 13, respectively.

SUBTALAR COMPLEX

Pathologic conditions involving the subtalar joint (STJ) can arise due to abnormal biomechanics, fixed pathology, arthritides, and trauma (Table 1). Articulation between the calcaneus and talus has been called the "torque converter" of the foot because of its important biomechanical influence on the other joints of the foot.

Os Trigonum Syndrome

The os trigonum is an accessory bone that forms when the ossification center for the lateral tubercle of the talus fails to fuse with the body of the talus. Usually the anomaly is seen on routine lateral x-rays of the foot. However, this accessory bone may become pinched between the calcaneus and the tibia, leading to pain above the calcaneus at the posterior ankle joint. The condition is usually seen in ballet dancers. A physical exam may reveal direct tenderness in the posterior ankle or pain with ankle joint range of motion. Pain can be reproduced by palpating medial and

deep to the peroneal tendons. It is important to rule out fracture of the lateral tubercle by evaluation of a lateral x-ray of the foot and ankle.

Conservative treatment may include NSAIDs, strapping, and physical therapy. If these fail, surgical excision of the accessory bone through a posterolateral incision is indicated.

Sinus Tarsi Syndrome

Inflammation within the sinus tarsi secondary to trauma or overuse can lead to a painful condition called sinus tarsi syndrome. Chronic inversion ankle sprains are a common etiology.

Pain can be elicited by directly palpating the sinus tarsi on the lateral aspect of the rear foot. There will also be pain upon inversion and eversion of the STJ. The condition may be difficult to differentiate from a tear or sprain of the anterior talofibular ligament.

Treatment includes injection therapy, NSAIDs, orthotics, taping/strapping, and physical therapy. Oblique radiographs or a computed tomographic (CT) scan should be taken to rule out fracture or arthritis of the STJ.

Arthritides

Degenerative joint disease, rheumatoid arthritis, and gout may affect the subtalar joint (see Chapter 15). Posttraumatic arthritis of the STJ is common following calcaneal fractures, especially if they are intra-articular. Many of these patients require triple arthrodesis.

ANKLE

The ankle is a key focal point in the transmission of body weight during ambulation and bears more weight per unit area than any other joint in the body. It is capable of adjustments necessary for fine balance on a wide variety of terrain. Its integrity depends on the paradoxical function of stability and mobility. Because the joint is subject to the concentrated stress associated with standing as well as movement, the ankle is often involved in static and dynamic deformities. In fact, injuries to the ankle joint, the majority of which are seen by primary care physicians, are the most common conditions encountered in treatment of athletic injuries. The prevalence of such injuries has been variously estimated to be between 10 and

TABLE 1. *Pathology of the Subtalar Joint*

I. Biomechanical (Chapter 12)
  A. Excessive STJ pronation leading to pes planus and its related foot pathology
  B. Excessive STJ supination leading to pes cavus and its related foot pathology.

II. Fixed Pathology
  A. Coalition (Chapter 10)
  B. Varus/valgus (Chapter 2)
  C. Congenital vertical talus
  D. Os trigonum syndrome

III. Arthridites
  A. Degenerative joint disease (Chapter 15)
  B. Gout (Chapter 14)
  C. Rheumatoid arthritis (Chapter 15)
  D. Sinus tarsi syndrome
  E. Posttraumatic syndrome

IV. Trauma (Chapter 13)
  A. Calcaneal fractures
  B. Talar fractures

90%, with the highest rate occurring among basketball players. At least one study has estimated the incidence to be one significant ankle sprain per day per 10,000 population. Furthermore, ankle injuries are not always minor and may be associated with prolonged disability and recurrent instability in 25–40% of patients for several months to several years. Therefore, a casual approach (e.g., "It is only a sprain") to the diagnosis and management of these injuries is not tenable. The ubiquitous and unpredictable nature of ankle injuries mandates a precise understanding of the mechanism of injury, a clear ability to assess the degree of damage, and a solid understanding of appropriate treatment modalities in the acute and rehabilitative phases.

General Pathogenetic Mechanisms of Injury

Most ankle trauma frequently involves both ligamentous and bony damage. A number of anatomic factors contribute to such a combination injury. Ankle mortise asymmetry creates inherent instability during inversion. The longer lateral malleolus provides a mechanical barrier to eversion ligamentous injury due to its greater surface contact with the talus. In addition, the dome of the talus is appreciably wider anteriorly than posteriorly. During inversion and plantar flexion, the narrow posterior aspect of the talus occupies proportionately less space within the mortise. As a result, the increased ankle joint play, together with the inherent block to eversion, creates predominantly lateral stress forces. Additional complicating factors include a tight heel cord and deficient proprioception. Many athletes, particularly females, have tight heel cords that force heel inversion. Regular walking on smooth, flat surfaces leads to a proprioceptive deficiency that is aggravated on irregular, rough playing surfaces. Finally, the lateral ligaments of the ankle are smaller and weaker than the medial deltoid ligament.

Nonanatomical factors such as surface configuration and footwear are often responsible for injury. Irregular surfaces, particularly those with holes, can produce obvious damage to the ankle. Less obvious circumstances such as banked tracks can lead to repetitive ankle trauma and long-term ankle disability. Finally, defective, old, or inappropriately fitted footwear can result in inversion or eversion stress.

Clinical Evaluation

The following items should be carefully investigated in taking a history in all ankle injuries.

1. What were the position of the foot and the direction of stress when the injury occurred (e.g., eversion, inversion, flexion, extension, or a combination)?

2. Was there immediate disability, or did symptoms occur at a later time?

3. At the time of injury, were any snaps, pops, or crunches noted?

4. When and to what degree were pain, swelling, and discoloration noted?

5. Were there any preexisting problems associated with the joint (e.g., previous injury or systemic disease)?

6. Was medical care sought? What did the evaluation show? Was treatment initiated, and, if so, what were the results?

7. Did the injury occur acutely or from overuse?

8. What is the functional capacity of the joint at present?

9. What were the surface conditions at the time of injury?

As a final comment, it should be understood that a careful history also usually identifies the site of pathology and the severity of tissue trauma. There are situations, however, when a misdiagnosis can result. For specific types of ankle trauma, consult Chapter 13.

BIBLIOGRAPHY

1. Amis J, Jennings L, Graham D, et al: Painful heel syndrome: Radiographic and treatment assessment. Foot Ankle 9:91–95, 1988.
2. Baxter DE, Pfeffer GB, Thigpen M: Chronic heel pain: Treatment rationale. Orthop Clin North Am 20:563–570, 1989.
3. Kwong PK, Kay D, Voner RT, White MW: Plantar fasciitis: Mechanics and pathomechanics of treatment. Clin Sports Med 7:119–126, 1988.

Chapter 10

PEDIATRICS

Stuart Plotkin, D.P.M., and
Michael P. DellaCorte, D.P.M.

EMBRYOLOGY

Much foot pathology can be related to intrauterine development. The lower limb buds start to form at the end of the fourth week, just slightly after the upper extremities. As ontogeny recapitulates phylogeny, the lower extremity follows the development of our cold-blooded forebearers, with the foot being in the same plane as the leg, not perpendicular. During the eighth week, ossification begins, and a critical rotation takes place. The upper extremity rotates 90 degrees outward, placing the palms forward. The lower extremity rotates inward by the same amount, placing the soles posteriorly. A developmental overrotation leads to in-toe gait.

By the ninth week, the metatarsals continue to be adducted, but the calcaneus, which up to this time was adjacent to the talus, begins to migrate plantarly. The ankle joint develops its articulation with the talus. The foot is still parallel to the leg and inverted. During the next few weeks, the ankle dorsiflexes, and the degree of inversion starts to decrease due to bony torsional change in the calcaneus and talar neck. If this does not fully resolve, a permanent rearfoot and forefoot varus may occur. The lower extremity can be visualized with diagnostic ultrasound by week 10, and the foot by week 24 (Figs. 1 and 2). Many congenital deformities can be diagnosed at this time, including spina bifida, neural tube defects, clubfoot, amelia, phocomelia, achondroplasia, anencephaly, dwarfism, osteogenesis imperfecta, rocker-bottom feet, and polydactyly. Early diagnosis is important, because some deformities may be linked to or indicative of significant, if not life-threatening, medical disorders. Clubfoot and renal agenesis have such a link.

EXAMINATION OF THE LOWER EXTREMITY

As much as 70% of the adult population will eventually suffer from foot ailments as a result of untreated congenital problems. These include disabling deformities such as bunions, hammer toes, heel spurs, and degenerative arthritis. Many of these disabilities can be prevented if structural and functional biomechanical faults are detected and treated early. It is a common misconception that many pediatric gait abnormalities are outgrown. It is another serious misconception that if pain is not involved, there is no reason to treat. It is actually rare that pediatric patients complain of frank pain. Their symptoms are much more subtle. Tripping and falling, often asking to be carried, refusing to walk any distance, and lack of interest in sports are more common complaints. The importance of early diagnosis and treatment cannot be overemphasized.

In examining a joint's range of motion, the examiner should take note of (1) symmetry with respect to the contralateral mate, (2) quality of motion, and (3) quantity (measured in degrees) and direction of motion, and should also determine if the noted deformities are structural (bony) or functional (soft tissue). Structural deformities tend to be more rigid and difficult to treat conservatively, whereas functional or positional deformities tend to

61

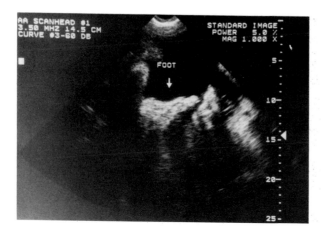

FIGURE 1. Ultrasound scan showing the foot.

be flexible, easily reducible, and more successfully treated.

Because all of the lower extremity joints function as a unit, all ultimately affect foot function in gait. Each joint must be individually examined. For instance, in-toe gait—a common complaint among children—often has a femoral component. Either soft tissue structures around the hip joint are limiting external rotation (functional) or there is an abnormal torque in the femur itself (structural). Torsional deformities (valgus, varus) of the tibia can also cause in-toe gait.

THE ANKLE JOINT

An infant's ankle can be dorsiflexed almost to the point at which the dorsal foot contacts the leg. There is up to 15 degrees of dorsiflexion in the adolescent. Twenty degrees is the normal value for plantarflexion. Limitation of dorsiflexion (i.e., equinus) is common and quite debilitating.

A child with limited ankle joint dorsiflexion demonstrates either a bouncy type of gait with an early or premature heel-off, flexed knees, or severe flatfoot. It is not uncommon for a very young child to walk occasionally on the toes, but this should resolve after 3–6 months. A severely pronated or flatfoot type of gait with everted heels should suggest an equinus deformity. In the older child, growth spurts may produce an equinus, as may muscle overdevelopment in an athletic child.

Treatment in the infant consists of passive stretching done by the parent. With the baby lying supine, the knees locked, and the foot slightly supinated, the parent can slowly dorsiflex the foot and hold it for 5 seconds. The exercise is repeated five times at every diaper change. The older child is best stretched by standing and facing a wall with elbows extended, hands on the wall, and one leg in

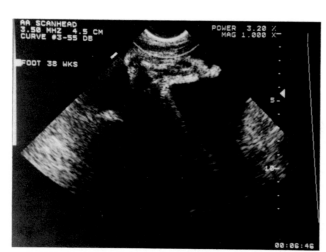

FIGURE 2. Ultrasound showing the foot at 38 weeks of gestation.

front of the other. Both legs should be slightly rotated internally. With the knees locked in extension and the heel flat on the ground, the child leans in toward the wall, bending elbows and the front knee. If done correctly, the child should feel a strong pulling behind the posterior knee. The position is held for 5 seconds and repeated five times without bouncing. If the pulling is only mild, the child should then step slightly farther from the wall. If no improvement is noted with this stretching exercise, a specialist should be consulted.

THE SUBTALAR JOINT (STJ)

In neonates, the STJ is not completely matured; the calcaneus is still in varus. In the young walker, the STJ is markedly pronated; there is a wide base of gait, the legs appear bowed, and the angle of the gait is high. If the angle of gait approaches zero degrees or becomes internal, it is considered pathologic, and a specialist should be consulted. By age 3 years, the child's gait is approaching maturity; however, the foot may remain pronated. By age 7, the STJ should no longer be excessively pronated. An overpronated foot should be treated.

Valgus Deformities

Planovalgus. Planovalgus (i.e., flat arch with an everted heel) is a congenital deformity that can be identified as early as at birth. All children generally walk with some degree of planovalgus, more appropriately called pronation. The differential diagnosis consists of idiopathic, calcaneovalgus, vertical talus, tarsal coalition, and biomechanical and ligamentous laxity. Vertical talus and tarsal coalition are rigid deformities; the others are flexible.

Calcaneovalgus. Calcaneovalgus is characterized by dorsiflexion and eversion of the entire foot and occurs in approximately one in 1,000 births. It is 1.6 times more common among females and is significantly more common among firstborns. It is believed to be caused by excessive uterine pressure. Examination of calcaneovalgus reveals a lack of plantarflexion and inversion. X-rays reveal normal bony architecture, normal articulation, and no subluxation. Calcaneovalgus is a positional deformity caused by contractures of the anterior and lateral muscle groups. If the deformity is significant (not easily reducible by

manipulation) and left untreated, an unstable pronated foot is often the result.

In mild to moderate deformities, treatment consists of manipulation and stretching by the parent, best accomplished by gently inverting and plantarflexing (supinating) the foot. The contracted soft tissue structures should be stretched and held for a count of 5 seconds and repeated 10–20 times. A convenient situation for performing these exercises is every time the diaper is changed. For more significant deformities, stretching and manipulation followed by plaster casting are recommended. The casts are generally changed every 7–10 days and should be applied by a specialist. After the deformity is reduced, bivalve casts or special shoes should be used to maintain the correction.

Congenital Vertical Talus

Vertical talus, also known as rocker-bottom foot or convex pes valgus, is a dorsolateral dislocation of the talocalcaneal navicular joint. The navicular articulates with the dorsal neck of the talus, locking it in a vertical and plantarflexed position. It is a rare deformity often associated with important neuromuscular diseases, including myelomeningocele and arthrogryposis multiplex. There are significant anomalies in the body of the calcaneus, talus, and navicular, in addition to secondary contractions of ligaments and tendons.

Clinically, the sole of the foot is convex, with the apex being the bulge of the talar head plantarly. The forefoot is dorsiflexed and abducted, and the hindfoot is plantarflexed. The anterior and lateral muscle groups are contracted, and the navicular may be prominent dorsally. The diagnosis can be confirmed radiographically in the newborn, despite the fact that the navicular has not yet ossified. The severely plantarflexed talus and the equinus position of the calcaneus are pathognomonic. Because it is a rigid deformity, it is not significantly improved by conservative means. Despite the fact that the young child may not complain of pain, his or her gait will be unstable and will lead to significant soft tissue and arthritic pathology early in life. Swift diagnosis and surgical correction are required.

FLATFOOT

Flatfoot is the term used to indicate absence of the normal arch. The incidence of flatfoot is approximately 30–40 per 100 children aged 1.5–3 years due to the large amount of plantar fat. The rate decreases to about 4 per 100 in older children and adults. The deformity can be flexible (arch present off weight bearing, absent on weight bearing) or rigid (arch absent off weight bearing and on weight bearing). The deformity can also be painful or asymptomatic. Excessive pronation is the most common cause of flexible flatfoot and is generally normal up until age 6 years. After that age it is considered abnormal. Rigid flatfoot deformities are usually caused by muscle spasm, bone adaptation, or trauma.

Flexible Flatfoot

Biomechanical abnormalities, leading to excessive pronation, are the most common causes of flexible flatfoot (see Chapter 12). A comprehensive biomechanical exam of the lower leg identifies the causative segment (e.g., tight heel cord, calcaneal varus) (see Chapter 2). Symptoms vary from asymptomatic to severe pain upon ambulation, and treatment is geared to the affected segment and the symptoms. Os tibiale externum, an accessory bone found medial to the navicular, is another cause of flexible flatfoot and is present in approximately 2–10% of the population. It is invested in the posterior tibial tendon, weakening the tendon's ability to support the medial arch in gait due to the fact that the tendon attaches more medially rather than plantarly. The force vector, therefore, becomes more adductory rather than supportive. Clinically, the non-weight-bearing foot has a normal range of motion in appearance, but on weight bearing, the foot collapses and pronates maximally. The calcaneus everts, and a significant medial protrusion can be noted by the navicular. The protrusion may be inflamed by shoe irritation, causing a painful adventitious bursitis and a posterior tibial tendinitis. Treatment in this case generally involves surgical excision of the accessory bone and advancement of the posterior tibial tendon.

For children aged 3 and under, an asymptomatic flexible flatfoot requires no treatment. In severe flatfoot deformities and in mildly symptomatic flatfeet, a medial Thomas heel may be added to the shoe. In symptomatic toddlers, a stabilizing orthotic that cups the heel may be used to prevent severe eversion of the calcaneus. For children aged 3–8 years, a moderate to severe flatfoot should be treated regardless of symptomatology because of possible adult sequelae (e.g., bunions, hammer toes, fasciitis). Proper treatment consists of passive stretching of any contracted muscle (facilitated by parents twice daily for 10–15 minutes), proper-fitting shoes, and a functional orthotic. Heel wedges may also be used. For the symptomatic child (e.g., with associated tendinitis, bursitis), conservative treatment consists of nonsteroidal anti-inflammatory drugs (NSAIDs), ice, rest, elevation, and immobilization. An orthotic may reduce symptoms caused by an unstable overpronated foot and shoe irritation by controlling adduction and plantar flexion of the talus. If symptoms do not improve in three to six months, a specialist should be consulted. After age 8, the child may be treated as an adult, with an orthotic that has appropriate forefoot and rearfoot posts. The prognosis gets progressively better the earlier treatment is started. Reduction of symptoms and muscle contractures, improved joint range of motion, lessening eversion of the calcaneus in gait, and better stability are important criteria to assess biannually.

It is important to note that arch integrity is determined by the shape and articulation of the tarsal bones. Muscles are not involved in maintaining arch height. It is, therefore, futile to try to improve the arch height by various exercises. Picking up pencils, moving marbles with the toes, and other arch-strengthening exercises should be abandoned. The archaic technique of encasing the flatfoot in orthopedic rigid shoes should also be discontinued.

Rigid Flatfoot

Peroneal spastic flatfoot is a painful deformity usually caused by a tarsal coalition. Tarsal coalition is generally not apparent at birth. Coalitions are defined as either osseous, cartilaginous, or fibrous bridges between two tarsal bones. The two most common coalitions involve the talocalcaneal medial and posterior facets (Fig. 3) and the calcaneonavicular joint (Fig. 4). Fusions involving other tarsal bones have been identified and are quite rare. Clinically, many coalitions are not symptomatic in the young child but may present in the second decade of life as the coalition begins to limit joint motion and the child reaches puberty. Complaints of leg pain exacerbated by activity are frequent. The most common physical finding is limitation of subtalar joint (STJ) motion. Often peroneal spasms are

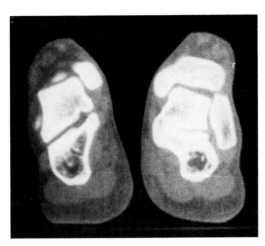

FIGURE 3. CT scan showing tarsal coalition of medial facet.

caused by the body's attempt to splint the painful segment. Fibrous coalitions tend to allow the greatest motion; cartilaginous and osseous bars create less motion and more symptoms. Conventional x-rays may not demonstrate the bar, but magnetic resonance imaging and computerized tomography scans are useful.

If diagnosis is not made early, there are secondary signs of talocalcaneal coalition that are actually caused by lack of STJ motion. The most striking changes consist in talar breaking, broadening of the lateral process of the talus, and narrowing and slanting of the posterior facet of the talus.

Treatment is geared to the severity of the symptoms. For mild discomfort, NSAIDs and rest may be all that are required. For moderate discomfort due to peroneal spasms, a common peroneal nerve block may be required followed by a below-the-knee cast, with the STJ held in the neutral position. After six weeks, this should be followed by a functional orthotic with specialized posting to control subtalar joint motion. If conservative treatment plans fail, surgical excision of the calcaneonavicular bar with interposition of soft tissue is required. Talocalcaneal bars are more difficult to treat, and surgical correction remains controversial.

IN-TOE

In-toe or in-toeing is defined as one or both feet pointing toward the midline of the body. The ambulating and nonambulating infant may show signs of in-toeing that can be identified and treated early. A family history, including any delivery complications or developmental changes, is important. Questions about older siblings can supply invaluable information concerning the possible end results. A sibling's outgrowing of a similar problem increases the likelihood that a physiologic delay in maturation will resolve. The level of the parents' concern should also be assessed and considered in the treatment plan.

A systematic segmental biomechanical examination will determine the level of the deformity (see Chapter 2). Multilevel deformities are quite common (Table 1). In the walking child, examination of the gait can direct the practitioner to diagnosis of the appropriate level. The angle of gait can be approximated visually or by the use of a paper track and powdered chalk or ink system. If the patella is deviated medially, the segment involved is probably the femur or hip joint. With the patella in the frontal plane, a tibial or STJ segmental deformity is likely. If only the distal foot is deviated, a metatarsus adductus deformity can be suspected. It is also important to determine if the involved segment is causing a structural

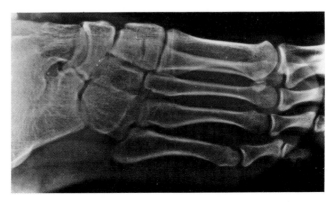

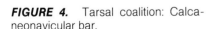

FIGURE 4. Tarsal coalition: Calcaneonavicular bar.

TABLE 1. *Causes of In-toe Gait from Proximal to Distal*

Proximal	Internal femoral position
	Femoral anteversion
	Pseudolack of knee
	Internal tibial torsion
Distal	Metatarsus adductus

or positional deformity. Treatment must be directed to the specific level of the deformity.

Most positional, as opposed to structural, in-toe deformities (Table 1) are easier to treat, and they resolve with greater success. The decision to treat can be a difficult one. Does one wait for physiologic correction to take place? How can one determine to what degree the deformity will spontaneously resolve? What symptoms are present and what can be expected? How much disability will the deformity cause? What are the risk factors of the treatment plan? How concerned are the parents? It is necessary to determine the risk versus the benefit of the treatment. If the treatment is easily tolerated and carries little iatrogenic risk, initiating treatment is reasonable. The consequences of waiting and watching will be worse than treating a patient who may have undergone spontaneous correction. The vast number of adults with disabling foot pathology (e.g., chronic ankle sprains, hammer toes, bunions, and degenerative joint disease) is, in itself, confirmation.

The cornerstone of any treatment plan is mobilization of the affected part. The treatment of choice of in-toed gait originating above the knee involves a new device—the Counter Rotational Splint, marketed by Langer Biomechanics Group for about $100 (The Langer Biomechanics Group, Inc., 11 East Industry Court, Deer Park, NY 11729). Its many advantages include attachability to any standard shoe, easy sizability, adjustability to precise angles, and acceptability by child and parent. It protects the vulnerable subtalar and midtarsal joints from excessive pronation. Most important, it allows complete freedom of independent leg motion in all directions except internal rotation. Its dynamic motion and enhanced patient compliance increase the success rate. It is indicated for children up to age 4, after which orthotics are used to manage in-toe gait.

Controversy has arisen over the use of rigid bars across the feet (e.g., Denis Brown bar) to treat in-toe secondary to rotational disorders of the leg. Some practitioners state that since many children outgrow this problem, any treatment is unnecessary. Others worry that damage may be done to the distal joints, that is, STJ, ankle, and knee. Because the philosophy of treatment is to ensure that the treatment is not worse than the disease, gentle guidance that assists normal development rather than forced stress on the lower extremity joints is recommended. The bar should, therefore, be used only at night to eliminate the prone in-toe position. If the Denis Brown bar is used, it is important that it be bent 5–10 degrees so that the feet are inverted and the STJ is protected from excessive pronatory forces. It is common today to see adults with significant pathology resulting from improper use of the Denis Brown bar. An iatrogenic flatfoot is a good example of the cure being worse than the illness. The connecting bar length should be approximately equal to or slightly greater than the distance between the anterior superior iliac spines. When correction is achieved, it is essential to continue its use to prevent relapse; the general rule is to continue treatment for at least half again the time it took to correct the deformity. It is important to remove the device during the day in order to mobilize and stretch the joints. In the walking or crawling child, it should be used only as a night splint. Initiating treatment as early as possible is imperative.

If the in-toeing is originating at the hip joint, the parent is instructed to hold the femur firmly above the knee and gently hold the foot. The femur is externally rotated with the hand holding the femur. It is important not to apply pressure to the foot, because the STJ and knee joints will be strained. The hip joint is held firmly at the end of its external range of motion for a count of five, then relaxed. The exercise should be repeated five times per affected leg, a few times a day. Also helpful is to change the child's sitting pattern from sitting with the feet underneath, or in a W position, to one with the legs outstretched. Prone sleeping with the legs internal should be discouraged. Ice skating, roller skating, and ballet are sports that may help to reduce the deformity in older children.

If the in-toe gait is originating from decreased tibial torsion (i.e., reduced amount of bony torque in the tibia/fibula), treatment options are limited. Although the deformity is often outgrown, a full 10% of cases will not resolve. Problems develop when the patient tries to compensate for the in-toe gait by actively pronating the foot. STJ pronation allows the forefoot to abduct, decreasing the appearance of in-toed gait. Tripping and falling symptoms occur from pronatory compensation on an unstable foot. Sometimes one foot catches the other in gait. Treatment with an orthotic device is directed toward achieving normal foot function. Parents should be advised that reducing compensatory pronation will make the child appear more in-toed. The symptoms, however, will lessen.

METATARSUS ADDUCTUS

Deviation of the tarsometatarsal joints of the forefoot can cause in-toe gait. Metatarsus adductus is adduction of metatarsals 1–5 at the tarsometatarsal joint. There may also be an associated varus or inverted relationship between the metatarsals and the lesser tarsus (i.e., adductovarus). The etiology remains unclear. One theory argues that there is a delayed fetal maturation of the forefoot. Other etiologic theories include intrauterine crowding, genetic components, and abnormal muscle activity. The incidence of metatarsus adductus is greater than 1 per 1,000 births.

Clinically, there are forefoot adduction, separation between the hallux and the lesser toes, and a C-shaped foot. Another common finding is abnormal pull of the abductor hallucis as well as of the anterior and posterior tibial muscles, which may be due to an abnormal innervation or insertion. The child should be examined sitting and walking, age permitting. It is important to determine the flexibility of the deformity by holding the rearfoot immobile with one hand and abducting the forefoot on the rearfoot. If the deformity can be manually reduced, treatment will be significantly easier. It is important to note the lateral column of the foot (i.e., the fifth metatarsal and the cuboid articulation). If this is straight or can be straightened, treatment will be significantly better.

Although many foot bones have not yet completely ossified by infancy, an x-ray can be beneficial for determining the severity of the deformity and for following the progress of bony improvement. On x-ray evaluation, a heel bisector line should pass through or near the second toe. If it passes lateral to the third toe, metatarsus adductus is present. A significant deformity shows the heel bisector's passing through the fourth toe laterally. Metatarsus adductus can be differentiated from

talipes equinovarus by the appearance of a normal rearfoot and normal talocalcaneal angle on x-ray. It is common for the first metatarsal to have a greater deviation from the heel bisector than the lesser metatarsals. If only the first metatarsal is affected, it is designated a metatarsus primus adductus.

It is vital to initiate treatment as soon as possible, especially before the child begins walking. In addition, it is important to note that, if a patient is merely watched until the time when it is apparent that the deformity will not be outgrown, successful treatment will be very difficult, if not impossible. The sequelae of untreated metatarsus adductus are increased risk of bunion deformities, excessive pronation, and difficulty in fitting shoe gear.

If the cause of the in-toed gait lies solely in the foot, as in metatarsus adductus, the treatment must be directed to that segment alone. In the infant, this deformity is generally very flexible. With a slight abductory force on the fifth metatarsal head, the forefoot can be placed in its corrected position. If the deformity is mild to moderate, it can be treated with stretching exercises alone. The parent is instructed to hold the heel firmly with one hand, and place lateral pressure on the first metatarsal head, being careful to avoid pressure on the hallux. The forefoot is then abducted and held to a count of five. It is vital that the STJ not pronate while the forefoot is abducted. This exercise is performed five times per affected foot during each diaper change.

The treatment of choice in severe yet flexible metatarsus adductus has traditionally been serial plaster casts. This remains an excellent treatment plan but has been replaced by cleaner and less psychologically disturbing (to the parent) techniques. The technique for using serial plaster casts requires several minutes of initial mobilization of the forefoot. The foot and leg are well padded with cast liner (e.g., Webril). A 2 inch, extra-fast-setting plaster roll is immersed in water and rolled onto the foot, starting exactly at the metatarsal heads. The toes are avoided. The plaster is quickly rolled onto the leg. Some practitioners recommend above-the-knee casting with flexed knee, but most feel that a below-the-knee cast is sufficient. An assistant is often required to hold the baby or the plaster. The cast should not be rubbed in well, so as to allow for easy removal by the parent. Most important, after the cast is applied, the rearfoot is held in

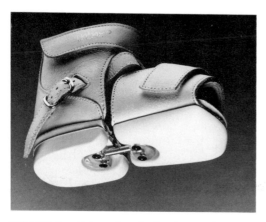

FIGURE 5.   Bebax shoe for treatment of metatarsus adductus.

neutral position and only the forefoot is abducted. The STJ must not be allowed to pronate, as this may cause an iatrogenic flatfoot. The cast is changed every 7 to 10 days and is best removed by the parent the night before by soaking in dilute vinegar and unrolling. A cast cutter should be avoided due to its frightening noise. Often four to six casts are applied before correction is achieved. The earlier that treatment is initiated, the faster the resolution. Once the correct position has been achieved, it is necessary to maintain it with a night splint to decrease the possibility of relapse. Radiographs and ink imprints should be used to track clinical progress.

Two new devices have been marketed recently: the Bebax shoe (Fig. 5) and the Wheaton brace (Fig. 6). The Bebax shoe has separate rearfoot and forefoot sections, connected by two multidirectional swivel joints. It can be adjusted in all three body planes to correct for metatarsus adductus or varus. The exact angulation is set by the practitioner. The device is easily tolerated, is less threatening to the parent, and, most important, allows for daily manipulation. It is also useful postoperatively to maintain correction and is an excellent night splint after serial casting. It maintains the STJ in neutral while applying pressure to the forefoot.

The Wheaton brace is a thermoplastic splint designed to maintain the STJ in its neutral position while applying an abductory force to the forefoot (Fig. 7). In the past, splints have been ineffective in treating metatarsus adductus due to their inability to immobilize the rearfoot and so have been used mostly to maintain postoperative or postcasting correction. The Wheaton brace has the ability to correct the deformity with fewer complications and emotional grief. It is also well tolerated and allows for daily manipulation. It is recommended for children aged 2–8 months, thus making early diagnosis imperative.

In the older child with flexible metatarsus adductus, the above modalities are poorly tolerated. A straight-last shoe with medial heel wedge to protect the STJ, in addition to stretching exercises, may be useful. The older techniques of reversing shoes and using reverse-last or pronator shoes must be abandoned. These unquestionably cause damage to the STJ, leading to flatfoot or skew foot. By the same token, a Denis Brown bar is completely ineffective for treatment of metatarsus adductus.

Serial below-the-knee casts are used to treat rigid deformities. Surgical intervention should be considered if the problem does not resolve in several months.

CAVUS FOOT

The high-arched, or cavus, foot type in many ways is the mirror image of the flexible flatfoot. It is a rigid functioning foot unable to adapt to variations in terrain, prone to ankle sprains, and lacking in good shock absorption. A child with a cavus foot should elicit a high index of suspicion for neuromuscular disease. A neurologic workup and complete spine x-rays are imperative. Whereas a percentage of cases are simply idiopathic with

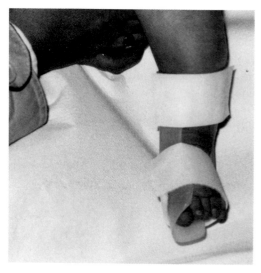

FIGURE 6.   Wheaton brace.

no pathologic cause, a great many can be traced to underlying neuromuscular disease. The differential diagnosis includes Charcot-Marie-Tooth disease, Dejerine-Sottas syndrome, Friedreich's ataxia, cerebral palsy, muscular dystrophy, polio, myelomeningocele, trauma, and tumor.

In appearance, the cavus foot demonstrates an excessively high arch, forefoot equinus, and often a fixed rearfoot varus. The deformity is progressive with contractures of the digits and atrophy of the plantar fat pad. There is great debate over the exact etiology, but most agree there is an imbalance of intrinsic and extrinsic musculature, including weakness and spasticity. Treatment must be directed to the neurologic causes but may include orthotic devices, stretching exercises, soft tissue surgical releases, and bony procedures if the deformity is fixed.

CLUBFOOT (TALIPES EQUINOVARUS)

The characteristics of talipes equinovarus (TEV) (Fig. 8) are an adducted forefoot, inverted rearfoot, equinus, and subluxation of the talocalcaneal navicular joints. There is a medial rotation of the entire foot around the talus. The navicular is medial to the talus and, in fact, almost abuts the medial malleolus. It is thought that the primary deformity is in the talar neck. Secondary changes are subluxation of the tarsal joints and soft tissue contractures, including the triceps, posterior tibial, flexor digitorum longus, and flexor hallucis longus muscles.

TEV can be clinically divided into two groups—rigid and flexible. The rigid deformity is more common and is characterized by exhibiting a true anomaly in the talar neck, subluxation of joints, leg atrophy, and a deep skin furrow across the medial heel and ankle. The skin is stretched so tight as to obliterate the normal skin lines on the dorsolateral aspect of the foot. This type of deformity is usually treated surgically. Flexible TEV is probably caused by intrauterine crowding and has no bony anomalies. There are no joint subluxations, atrophy, or deep skin furrows, and it is relatively easy to correct the deformity with manipulation and casting.

Common radiographic findings in TEV include reduction in the talocalcaneal angle almost to the point of superimposition of the talus on the calcaneus. An angle of less than 15 degrees is significant. Another useful

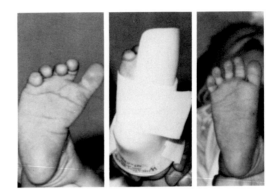

FIGURE 7. Metatarsus adductus before, during, and after treatment with Wheaton brace.

measure is the angle made by bisection through the long axis of the first metatarsal and bisection of the talus. Normally it should be between 0 and 15 degrees. An angle greater than 15 degrees indicates a medial subluxation of the talonavicular joint. X-rays should be taken in a relaxed and corrected position. Serial x-rays are important to monitor the treatment plan and to check for the possibility of an iatrogenic rocker-bottom foot, which is a severe flatfoot deformity in which the calcaneus is plantarflexed and the midtarsal joint is subluxed with the forefoot dorsiflexed. The apex of the deformity is in the midfoot.

Treatment should begin within the first few days of life. Initially, conservative treatment should be instituted even in the rigid clubfoot, despite the probable need for future surgery. Manipulation is vital. For the pediatric patient, it is important to remember that ligaments and tendons may be stronger than

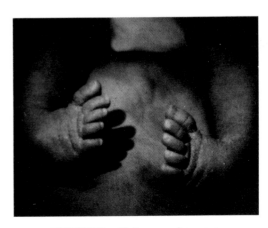

FIGURE 8. Talipes equinovarus.

the osteocartilaginous structures, so manipulation pressure should be gentle. Each segment is manipulated and corrected separately in the following order: metatarsus adductus, calcaneal varus, and equinus. The leg should be stabilized with one hand. The other hand is placed across the metatarsal plane with the thumb dorsal and lesser fingers plantar. The foot is distracted and gentle pressure applied to the talar head while pushing medially. The manipulation should be done for 10 minutes before casting. After manipulation, an above-the-knee cast should be applied. Once the metatarsus adductus is corrected, the calcaneal varus is addressed. Gentle eversion of the heel for 10 minutes is followed by an above-knee cast. After the calcaneus has been manipulated out of its varus position, the equinus can be corrected. It is important not to attempt reduction of the equinus initially or to dorsiflex the foot distal to the midtarsal joint (across the forefoot), because a midtarsal breach and a rocker-bottom foot may follow. With both thumbs, plantarly press on the distal calcaneus in a dorsiflexion direction. Exercise for 10 minutes, then apply an above-knee cast. The eventual goal is a foot with 10+ degrees of ankle dorsiflexion, a calcaneus that can evert past perpendicular, straight medial and lateral borders, and aligned talonavicular and talocalcaneal joints confirmed on x-ray.

At this point, the risk of relapse is great. Retention casting must be continued for 2–3 months followed by a splint such as the Bebax Shoe in which the physician can control the set angles. Reverse or pronator shoes are not recommended. If conservative measures fail, then surgical release is required.

JUVENILE BUNIONS

A common adult deformity, hallux abducto valgus, or bunion, can also be found in children. For generations, bunions were blamed on tight shoes. The science of the biomechanics of human gait has disproved this belief. Bunion formation is caused directly by an unstable forefoot, which in turn is caused by excessive STJ pronation. Due to the fact that this condition may include internal gait disorders, equinus, limb length inequality, varus or valgus foot, and leg deformities, a complete biomechanical evaluation is necessary. Most cases of symptomatic hallux abducto valgus become present in the older adult population

after decades of walking. The fact that some adolescents present with this deformity suggests that significant pronatory forces are acting on the foot. Although there may be a familial history of bunions, this should not be thought of as "a bunion gene" but rather as the inheritance of a foot structure that predisposes to excessive STJ pronation. For mild to moderate deformities, treatment should be directed at the biomechanical causes of excessive pronation. Only then can a correct functional orthotic be fabricated. Severe deformities require surgical intervention. A specialist should be consulted in these cases.

KOHLER'S DISEASE

Kohler's disease, or osteochondritis of the navicular, is common, particularly in 5- to 7-year-old boys. Clinically, it presents with pain over the navicular area. Kohler's disease may have a mechanical basis. The navicular is subject to great stress during locomotion and is one of the last bones to ossify. Radiographically, sclerosis and flattening of the navicular are diagnostic. Treatment again consists of rest, aspirin, orthotics, and, if necessary, a below-knee cast for 4–6 weeks. The course of the disease may take up to 18 months. The prognosis is good, but orthotics may have to be worn indefinitely.

SEVER'S DISEASE

Sever's disease, also called calcaneal apophysitis or osteochondrosis of the calcaneal apophysis, is a common cause of heel pain in active, stocky, 7- to 12-year-old boys. It is caused by excessive traction on the calcaneal apophysis by the Achilles tendon, particularly during running and jumping sports. Pain is elicited on palpation of the Achilles tendon insertion at the inferior heel surface. A tight Achilles tendon may predispose to the condition. X-rays are useful only in ruling out fracture or tumor. Normally, calcaneal apophysis ossification is irregular and dense and cannot be distinguished from an apophysitis. The differential diagnosis includes Achilles bursitis and tendinitis. Treatment consists of rest, ice, compression, elevation, elimination of jumping sports, shock-absorbing heel lifts such as sorbothane, and Achilles stretching exercises to 20 or 30 degrees. In severe cases, a below-knee cast may be used for 4–6 weeks. The prognosis is good, with resolution of the problem expected in the early teens.

SHOE GEAR

Shoe gear remains a controversial subject. In the prewalker, shoes are not recommended except for protection from the environment. In the beginning walker, a shoe with a sturdy heel counter and a shank flexible enough to bend under the child's weight is advised. Such a shoe holds the heel vertical and counteracts the physiologic excessive pronation that is due to lack of maturation. Running shoes (i.e., sneakers) made for toddlers are excellent in this regard. For the older child, the same criteria hold. The running shoe offers good shock absorption and control and is excellent for accommodating a functional orthotic when needed.

BIBLIOGRAPHY

1. Crawford AH, Gabriel KR: Foot and ankle problems. Orthop Clin North Am 18:649–666, 1987.
2. Drvaric DM, Kuivila TE, Roberts JM: Congenital clubfoot: Etiology, pathoanatomy, pathogenesis and changing spectrum of early management. Orthop Clin North Am 29:641–648, 1989.
3. Ganley J (ed): Podopediatrics. Clinics in Podiatry, vol. 1, no. 3. Philadelphia, W.B. Saunders, 1984.
4. Killam PE: Orthopedic assessment of young children: Developmental variations. Nurse Pract 14:27–30, 1989.
5. Lovell WW, Winter RB: Pediatric Orthopedics, Vols. 1 and 2. Philadelphia, J.B. Lippincott, 1986.
6. Phillips WA: The child with a limp. Orthop Clin North Am 18:489–502, 1987.
7. Staheli LT: Lower positional deformity in infants and children: A review. J Pediatr Orthop 10:559–563, 1990.
8. Staheli LT: Rotational problems of the lower extremities. Orthop Clin North Am 18:512–563, 1987.
9. Tachdjian MO: The Child's Foot. Philadelphia, W.B. Saunders, 1985.
10. Tax HR: Podopediatrics, 2nd ed. Baltimore, Williams & Wilkins, 1985.

Chapter 11

GERIATRICS

Michael P. DellaCorte, D.P.M., John Tsouris, D.P.M.,
and William F. Buffone, D.P.M.

Geriatric foot problems pose a special challenge to the primary care physician. In an era when average life expectancy is rising steadily, the need to identify and treat geriatric foot problems becomes a part of everyday practice. What may be a common foot problem or minor trauma to the middle-aged adult becomes a debilitating and sometimes crippling disorder in the elderly patient. Pain-free mobility is a major factor in the general well-being of the elderly, whereas foot problems are frequently associated with immobility. A normal geriatric foot is one that is asymptomatic and noncontributory to any mental, systemic, or local disorder. It has been estimated that 70% of the population over 65 years of age suffers from some kind of foot problem.

Factors contributing to the development of foot problems in the elderly include changes in gait, past foot care and management, hereditary problems, previous foot conditions that were not treated, emotional problems and changes in mental status, nutritional problems, systemic and local disease, hospitalization and confinement to bed, and various medications. Additional concerns and risk factors include increased susceptibility to infection, diabetes mellitus, other forms of neurovascular impairment, and atrophy associated with degenerative neuromuscular and musculoskeletal diseases. The most common podiatric complaints of the elderly are shown in Table 1. In addition to systemic disease, obesity and increased physical activity increase the incidence of foot ailments in the elderly.

CORNS AND CALLUSES

These lesions include heloma durum, heloma molle, heloma milliare, heloma vascularis, and tyloma. Although such conditions are common among all age groups, atrophy of the plantar fat pad, degenerative joint disease, and decreased pain threshold predispose the elderly to increased frequency of complaints. Commonly located dorsally on the digits (Fig. 1) and plantarly under the metatarsal heads (Fig. 2), these lesions are often accompanied by bursitis, capsulitis, or both. Abducted gait and shuffling are additional factors that generate increased stress and pressure on the soft tissues, leading to corns and calluses (Fig. 3).

A heloma molle is a heloma that develops between the toes. It is soft because it absorbs moisture from the interspace. This lesion typically forms over the medial aspect of the head of the proximal phalanx of the fifth toe or the lateral aspect of the base of the proximal phalanx of the fourth toe. Without treatment, the lesion may ulcerate and become infected. Conservative treatment involves both debridement of the lesion and padding to keep the toes separated. Surgical treatment of the fourth interspace soft corn is best achieved by resecting the head of the proximal phalanx of the fifth toe.

Corn and callus treatments range from debridement to surgery and are discussed in the general treatment guidelines section (see Chapter 20). Regarding surgery in the elderly, it should be noted that fear of surgery often outweighs the pain caused by the corn or

TABLE 1. *Common Foot Ailments in the Elderly*

Condition	Percentage of Elderly	Female-Male Ratio
Corns	20	4.7:1
Callus	12	2.6:1
Keratotic lesions	32	—
Toenail problems	24	1:1
Bunions and hammer toes	8	6:1
Swelling	—	2.5:1
Burning spells	—	2.9:1
Loss of feeling	—	1.8:1
Dry skin	4	2:1
Neurovascular and systemic	6.9	—
Ulcers	7	1:1

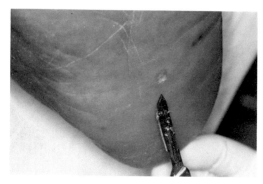

FIGURE 3. Plantar corn.

callus. Elderly patients should be made aware that long-standing helomas may progress to ulcerations or infections, making surgery mandatory and not elective.

TOENAIL PROBLEMS

Hypertrophy (Fig. 4) (thickening and hardening of the toenails) presents problems for the elderly patient with systemic disease, impaired vision, obesity, inability to bend, and/or loss of manual dexterity. Caused primarily by onychomycosis or impaired circulation left untreated, hypertrophy may result in subungual corns or ulcerations, infected ingrown toenails, and infections or ulcerations to adjacent toes. It may also lead to excessive pressure in shoe gear. The end result is painful, unstable

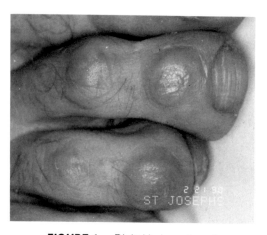

FIGURE 1. Digital heloma (corn).

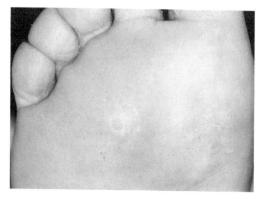

FIGURE 2. Plantar tyloma under the metatarsal head.

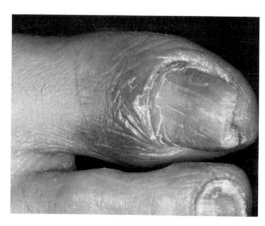

FIGURE 4. Thickening of the toenail.

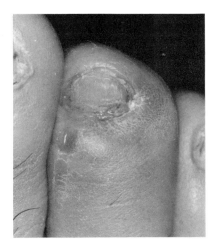

FIGURE 5. Onychocryptosis of a lesser digit.

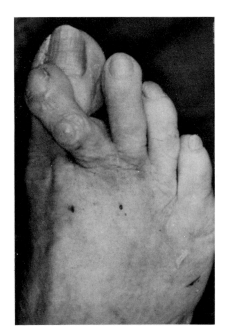

FIGURE 6. Mild bunion deformity with overlapping second digit.

ambulation. Treatment of nail disorders in the elderly should be as simple as possible, consisting of debridement or grinding.

Onychocryptosis (Fig. 5), or ingrown toenail, occurs when the free edge of the nail plate penetrates the periungual soft tissue. The etiology may be trauma, a diseased nail, an ill-fitting shoe, or improper cutting of the nail. A secondary infection may occur as may the formation of granulation tissue. Treatment is achieved by removing the offending nail spicule and granulation tissue, if present (see Chapter 20).

Onychogryposis, or ram's horn nails, are commonly seen in the elderly who have neglected their nail care (see Chapter 5). The skin edges and the eponychium surrounding these nails are very brittle in the elderly. Simple nail debridement may cause unintentional laceration to surrounding tissues. Combined with circulatory disorders, laceration may progress to infection. Documentation of the iatrogenic lesion along with a plan of care should be followed until the wound resolves.

Poor nutritional states lead to toenails that are atrophic, thin and brittle, and lackluster. Marked longitudinal ridges become prominent in these cases; this condition has been termed onychorrhexis. Treatment is geared toward nutritional counseling and local nail care.

HALLUX VALGUS

Bunion deformities (Figs. 6 and 7) in the elderly, accompanied by peripheral vascular disease, must be treated conservatively. Shoe

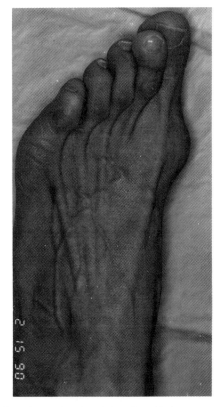

FIGURE 7. Bunion deformity with hammer toes.

gear needs to accommodate bony prominences, and custom-molded shoes may be required. Plaster cast impressions for molded shoes can be taken in the office by the primary care physician, or the patient can be referred to a specialist.

Physical therapy is another method of conservative treatment for bunions in the elderly. Care must be taken with heat and cold modalities in patients with neurologic or vascular impairments. If the patient is healthy enough, age should not be a criterion for foot surgery. Although surgery is geared toward relief of symptoms and not cosmesis in the elderly, foot surgery may increase mobility and add to the quality of life. A qualified foot surgeon should be consulted in these cases.

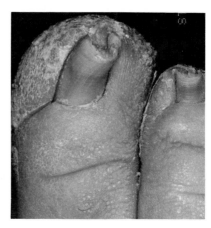

FIGURE 8. Dry, scaly skin—commonly seen in the elderly.

EDEMA

Chronic pedal edema secondary to cardiac, renal, hepatic, and vascular etiologies may lead to discomfort in shoe gear and alteration in gait patterns and mobility. Managing the cause medically, along with the use of support hose and elevation, should help to relieve symptoms.

BURNING

Burning sensations in the feet can be caused by a number of ailments such as biomechanic stress, neuroma, vascular disorders, diabetic and alcoholic neuropathies, and other systemic disorders such as hyperparathyroidism. Treatment is sometimes difficult and is geared to the underlying cause. When all else fails, physical therapy modalities such as cool whirlpool and transcutaneous electrical nerve stimulation may relieve symptoms.

XEROSIS

As aging progresses, there is a decrease in the amount of hydration of the skin, coupled with diminished sebaceous and eccrine activity, which leads to dry and scaly skin (Fig. 8). Dry skin can be prevented or improved by daily hydration of the affected areas. Bathing followed by the use of a topical emollient (e.g., a lanolin preparation) retards water loss. Hydration relieves itching and prevents fissuring that can lead to infection.

ULCERATIONS

Foot ulcerations are more common in the elderly. The type (Table 2) should be determined prior to treatment, because local ulcer care can promote injury and further functional loss, particularly with vascular and diabetic etiologies (Chapters 4, 16, and 18). The etiology of ulcerations comprises pressure, ischemia, and the neurotrophic, systemic, biomechanic, iatrogenic, patient-induced, or neoplastic diseases. It should be noted that ulcerations can appear to be a heloma or a tyloma. It is therefore necessary to debride all hyperkeratotic lesions prior to making a definitive diagnosis.

Treatment of ulcerations is generally a long process. If the primary etiology has been managed, weekly debridements and daily bandage changes (by the patient, the patient's family, or the home care nurse) are necessary. If the ulcers are infected, a culture and sensitivity should be taken by scalpel, not by swab, from the deepest area of the ulcer. Appropriate antibiotics should be administered in addition to local wound care (see Chapter 17). Local wound care of the ulcerations consists of debridement with a scalpel or tissue nipper. By use of an aseptic or sterile technique, all hyperkeratosis around the ulceration must be debrided. If the hyperkeratosis is allowed to cover over the ulceration, the epithelialization process will take much longer to complete, and the probability of infection is greater. The base of the ulceration should be debrided to a healthy bleeding level and then allowed to granulate. Wet to dry dressings of saline,

TABLE 2. *Lower Extremity Ulcers—Differential Diagnosis*

Types	Common Sites	Symptoms	Characteristics
Ischemic	Distal, dorsal digits Dorsal foot Lateral malleolar area	Severe pain Symptoms usually at night, relieved by dependency Trophic skin changes of chronic ischemia	Poor granulation tissue Poor color of tissue, possibly cyanotic, gray, black (gangrenous) Poor bleeding upon stimulation Irregular borders
Static	Lower third of leg, supramalleolar areas, particularly medially	Mild pain, relieved by elevation Edema of surrounding tissue Hyperpigmentation of surrounding skin	Granulating base Weeping edema Color: from red to cyanotic Mild bleeding on stimulation Shallow, irregular shape
Neurotrophic	Beneath pressure points or hyperkeratotic lesions (submetatarsal heads 1, 5, lateral fifth metatarsal base, dorsomedial navicular)	No pain—patient usually neuropathic Generally no surrounding edema	Punched-out lesions Red base, white rim Excellent bleeding

peroxide, or Betadine are applied between dressing changes. Dressings should be changed twice daily. DuoDerm Hydroactive dressings may also be used alone or in conjunction with the above debridements. Areas of devitalized tissue that cannot be debrided may be eliminated by the use of enzymes such as Elase.

Some ulcers are extremely painful, and the patient will not be able to tolerate aggressive debridements. In these cases, local anesthesia may be necessary along with oral pain medications for any postdebridement pain. The primary care physician should be cautious when trying the numerous ulcer dressings available. These dressings can sometimes cause maceration and infections and must be monitored on a daily basis.

PRESSURE ULCERS

Pressure ulcerations commonly occur in areas where bony prominences, in combination with insensitivity, lead to breakdown of overlying skin. Common sites in the foot of the geriatric patient are the skin overlying a hallux valgus, or hammer digit, the skin beneath a plantarflexed metatarsal head, the plantar aspect of the fifth metatarsal base, and the area overlying a prominent navicular tuberosity. The pressure may be from the shoe or simply from repetition of normal ambulation.

If the ulcer is caused by pressure or biomechanical problems, no matter how much debridement and local wound care is given, the ulcer will never resolve if weight is not dispersed from the affected area. Pressure

ulcers have been clinically classified into a four-grade system (Table 3) as follows: grade I occurs only at the epidermis; grade II involves all tissues to the subcutaneous fat layer; grade III extends through the fat to the fascia; and grade IV invades the fascia, bone, joints, and viscera. The amount of damage is often in the shape of an inverted cone. Molded shoes, dispersions with felt padding, and accommodative orthotics are the best modalities that the practitioner can use to eliminate or lessen the pressure to the affected area. Once the trauma or pressure has been eliminated, the ulcer is debrided as stated above.

Surgical debridement is indicated for nonhealing ulcers or ulcerations with wide areas of devitalized tissue, exposed tendon, or joint capsule. If bone is exposed in an ulceration, it is considered to be infected. Surgical intervention is then mandatory, and the patient should undergo surgical debridement of bone and surrounding soft tissue. A specialist should be consulted in these cases. The patient should be informed of the risks and consequences and the possible loss of digits, a foot, or a limb.

TABLE 3. *Classification of Pressure Ulcerations*

Grade	Clinical Appearance	Prognosis
I	Irregular soft tissue swelling and induration	Excellent
II	Shallow, full-thickness ulcer	Excellent
III	Deep ulcer into subcutaneous fat; foul smelling	Poor
IV	Deep ulcer with exposed bone, drainage, and necrosis	Poor

SKIN ATROPHY

Atrophy of the submetatarsal or subcalcaneal fat pads is a common geriatric cause of painful foot. The plantar aspect of the foot is naturally cushioned by fat. When this atrophies or reduces in size, the bony structures underlying the fat become much more prominent. Increased pressure is therefore placed on the bony prominences, causing pain. When such pain occurs under the plantar aspect of the metatarsal heads, it is called metatarsalgia. Tylomas, helomas, and bursitis are frequently the complaint. Diagnosis is made on clinical exam and evaluation. X-ray evaluation may be necessary to rule out underlying bone pathology. Treatment consists of gentle debridement of hyperkeratotic lesions, with padding for immediate relief. The skin is generally very thin and tears easily; therefore, the practitioner should be cautious with the use of adhesive pads or tape. Removal of the tape may tear the skin, causing further disability. Long-term relief can be accomplished by the use of soft tissue supplements, such as Spenco or Plastazote, that can be added to the foot orthotics or inserted directly into the shoe. Many sneakers available today have the soft tissue supplement already in place, and they may give the relief needed.

OSTEOPOROSIS

Osteoporosis is a condition caused by diminution of bone mass; it is very common in the elderly patient. After age 33, bone mass decreases, beginning earlier and proceeding more rapidly in women, until 20–40% of bone mass has been lost by the age of 65. The decrease in bone mass in women begins prior to menopause and is accelerated in the postmenopausal state. The rate and frequency of foot fractures therefore increase in aging persons, particularly women. It should also be noted that surgical procedures involving osteotomies should be carefully considered in the elderly with osteoporosis. Medical management of any underlying systemic cause of the osteoporosis and dietary counseling should be done. Evaluations every 6–8 months will help monitor the condition.

PAINFUL HEEL PAD SYNDROME

Heel pain is another common complaint in the elderly patient. Its primary etiology is atrophy of the subcalcaneal fat pad plus cumulative impact loading due to repetitive heel strike during walking. Once this natural cushion is gone, there ensues increased pressure on the inferior aspect of the calcaneus. Obesity, increased or prolonged ambulatory activity, hard floors or surfaces, and biomechanical abnormalities are the factors that predispose to the development of inferior calcaneal bursitis. The patient experiences pain upon ambulation, which is not immediately relieved by rest. Burning and throbbing may also occur.

Direct palpation produces tenderness in the central aspect of the heel proximal to the medial tubercle of the calcaneus, thus distinguishing this syndrome from a heel spur syndrome.

Conservative treatment includes rest, nonsteroidal anti-inflammatory drugs (NSAIDs), and dispersion padding (U pad) or an MF heel protector. The flexible heel protector is a tight-fitting piece of plastic that cups the heel and squeezes all the fat under the calcaneus, thus providing more cushioning. It should be used with a rubber sole wedge-type shoe. If this treatment is ineffective after 3–5 days, the calcaneal bursa should be injected (see Chapter 20). Up to four injections may be necessary to relieve symptoms and should be given weekly until symptoms subside. Physiotherapy modalities such as whirlpool and ultrasound may also be helpful. To prevent recurrence, shoe modifications with heel dispersion padding or foot orthotics with a calcaneal bursitis dispersion pad should be worn indefinitely.

PLANTAR FASCIITIS

As aging progresses, the muscles and ligaments supporting the bony structures of the foot weaken, causing a decrease in the calcaneal inclination angle and the metatarsal declination angle. This process puts extra stress on the plantar fascia, causing traction periostitis, or strain of the fascia fibers. Coupled with obesity, increased activity, and biomechanical abnormalities, acute plantar fasciitis can develop. The condition is more common in men than in women. The complaint usually consists of pain in the morning upon first weight bearing, which gradually gets better once ambulation continues. At rest, the fascia relaxes and shortens, but once full body weight is applied, the fascia is overstretched, causing pain that gradually resolves with sustained body weight and stretching. Chronic cases of fasciitis are painful all the time. Diagnostically, dorsiflexion of the digits stretches the fascia, causing pain, as does direct palpation of the anteromedial border of the calcaneal tuberosity. Treatment is discussed in Chapter 9.

ACHILLES TENDINITIS

The geriatric patient may suffer from Achilles tendinitis as a result of a chronic overuse situation in which an already less elastic soft tissue structure is subject to prolonged walking or standing. Direct shoe pressure at the Achilles insertion may also result in tendinitis. Not to be excluded are the more common causes such as a direct blow, a sudden forceful contraction, or metabolic and inflammatory etiologies such as gout or one of the arthritides. The condition presents with pain, erythema, and edema in the hindfoot proximal to the tendon insertion. Crepitation, nodules, or both may also be present, depending on the condition's chronicity. Management is discussed in Chapter 9. For a discussion of Achilles bursitis, see Chapter 9.

POSTERIOR TIBIAL TENDON DYSFUNCTION WITH RESULTANT PES PLANUS

Spontaneous strain, rupture, or degeneration of the posterior tibial tendon is acknowledged as one of the common causes of pes planus in middle-aged and geriatric patients. Acute valgus trauma (e.g., missing the rung of a ladder or a sudden step from a curb) results in loss of arch height as well as decreased ability to plantarflex and invert the foot. Pain along the tendon is a presenting symptom as is some instability in gait. The pain progresses and often becomes intractable. Physical findings verify loss of inversion and plantarflexion of the affected foot, with pain along the course of the tendon when attempting contraction against resistance. A defect may be noted, and it may be possible to sublux the tendon anteriorly. Conservative management of a dysfunctional posterior tibial tendon includes NSAIDs, a medial arch support, and an external medial buildup at the sole and heel. In problematic cases, surgical intervention with possible tendon repair may be necessary. For a discussion of this dysfunction relative to arthritis, see Chapter 15; to diabetes, see Chapter 16; and to the circulatory system, see Chapter 18.

SHOE GEAR

Shoe gear for the geriatric patient should have an upper made of a soft material. The sole should not be too firm and should have a good shock-absorbing heel. The insole should be well padded for support. Laced shoes are preferred to loafers, since they allow for swelling. For patients unable to tie shoelaces, Velcro closures are available. Depth inlay shoes allow insertion of orthotic or cushioning support. Molded shoes accommodate bony prominences. For patients who cannot afford or who refuse to wear molded shoes, running shoes (sneakers) may give some relief. A good running shoe has all of the above qualities, along with providing a feeling of youthfulness to the elderly.

BIBLIOGRAPHY

1. Albert SF, Jahnigen DW: Treating common foot disorders in older patients. Geriatrics 38:42–55, 1983.
2. Calkins E, Davis PJ, Ford AB (eds): The Practice of Geriatrics. Philadelphia, W.B. Saunders, 1986, pp 441–450.
3. Edelstein JE: Foot care for the aging. Phys Ther 68:1882–1886, 1988.
4. Gleckman RA, Czachor JS: Managing diabetes-related infections in the elderly. Geriatrics 44:37–46, 1989.
5. Helfand AE (ed): Clinical Podogeriatrics. Baltimore, Williams & Wilkins, 1981, pp 13–35.
6. Helfand AE: Nail and hyperkeratotic problems in the elderly foot. Am Fam Phys 39:101–110, 1989.
7. Jahss MH (ed): Disorders of the Foot, Vol. I. Philadelphia, W.B. Saunders, 1986, pp 964–977.
8. Mann RA (ed): DuVries Surgery of the Foot, 4th ed. St. Louis, C.V. Mosby, 1978, pp 401–409.
9. Yale JF: Yale's Podiatric Medicine, 3rd ed. Baltimore, Williams & Wilkins, 1987, pp 131–246.

Chapter 12

BIOMECHANICAL ABNORMALITIES

Karen A. Borsos, D.P.M.,
and Michael P. DellaCorte, D.P.M.

EQUINUS

If the ankle joint cannot obtain at least 10 degrees of dorsiflexion, the patient is said to have equinus (Fig. 1). The etiology can be congenital, adaptive, or a combination of both (Table 1).

There are three forms of compensation for equinus: uncompensated, partially compensated, and fully compensated. Compensation is possible at three joints of the foot: the midfoot, rearfoot, and forefoot. Compensation for equinus is first taken up by the midfoot through unlocking of the midtarsal joint (MTJ). If this unlocking cannot occur, the patient does not compensate. The heel "pops" off the ground very early during ambulation. With partial compensation, the foot pronates (arch flattening) at the midfoot, and the rearfoot (heel) leaves the ground early when walking. During full compensation, the forefoot pronates and allows the heel to leave the ground at the normal time when walking.

For treatment of acute Achilles tendinitis secondary to equinus, the patient should wear a higher-heeled shoe temporarily or a heel lift. Although this practice might worsen the patient's condition on a long-term basis, it eliminates acute symptoms over shorter periods. NSAIDs may also be helpful. For chronic gastrocnemius and gastrosoleus equinus, calf-stretching exercises increase ankle joint dorsiflexion. Functional foot orthoses, an excellent conservative treatment option for all types of equinus, are fabricated with the subtalar joint (STJ) in neutral position and are designed to prevent excess pronation. A heel lift, if the equinus is not due to a bony abnormality, is added to accommodate the equinus initially.

Then, in conjunction with exercises, the heel lift is gradually decreased until the equinus is resolved. For equinus deformities (e.g., spastic and ankle equinus) not responding to conservative therapy, surgery is another treatment option.

TRANSVERSE PLANE DEFORMITIES OF THE LOWER EXTREMITY

Several factors can cause abnormal angle of gait leading to abnormal gait cycle and associated foot problems. Any abnormality of the transverse plane of the lower extremity will affect the angle of gait. Pathology of the hip (congenital dislocation), femur (torsion), knee (ligamentous laxity), and tibia (torsion) can produce gait abnormalities. Hence, a thorough examination of the lower extremity, both static and dynamic, is essential in determining the level of abnormality causing the alteration in gait. If the hip, knee, leg, and ankle are normal, the abnormality exists in the foot.

FRONTAL PLANE DEFORMITIES OF THE FOOT

At birth, the calcaneus is inverted relative to the talus. The posterior surface of the calcaneus undergoes an external torsion that brings it in line with the talus. If this torsion does not occur, rearfoot varus is the result (see Chapter 10). Assessment is made by placing the STJ in a neutral position and noting its position relative to the longitudinal bisection of the posterior leg. Rearfoot valgus, a rare condition, occurs when there is too much torsion.

81

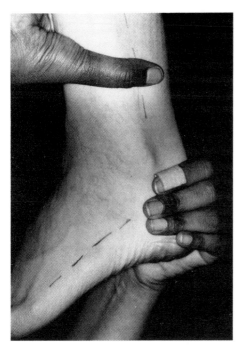

FIGURE 1.   Equinus: The lateral bisection of the leg is plantarflexed in relation to the lateral bisection of the foot.

Rearfoot Varus

Rearfoot varus is caused by any lower-extremity deformity that allows the heel to strike the ground with greater than 2 degrees of inversion. The patient can compensate either fully, partially, or not at all.

Uncompensated Rearfoot Varus

In uncompensated rearfoot varus, the foot strikes the ground inverted and stays inverted,

TABLE 1.   *Types of Equinus*

Type	Knee Joint	Dorsiflexion at the Ankle Joint
Gastrocnemius	Knee extended	<10°
	Knee flexed	>10°
Gastrosoleus	Knee extended	<10°
	Knee flexed	<10°
Ankle	Knee extended	<10°
	Knee flexed	<10°
Spastic	Observe gait	
	Calf muscle contraction leads to early heel-off	
Acquired	Calf muscle adapts to shortened position leading to early heel-off	

leading to a chronic inversion ankle sprain and rapid lateral shoe wear. The foot itself develops calluses along the lateral aspect of the heel and under the base of the fifth metatarsal. With the foot maintained in inversion, the peroneus longus muscle takes advantage of the rigid lateral column and plantarflexes the first ray, causing the patient to bear excess pressure on the tibial sesamoid. A hyperkeratotic lesion also develops below the first metatarsal. Hence, the patient with uncompensated rearfoot varus presents with a high arch, an inverted rearfoot, and a hyperkeratotic lesion of submetatarsal one and five. In addition, this patient is prone to inversion ankle sprains because the rearfoot maintains inversion. A painful heel may also be present owing to poor shock absorption.

Generally, conservative treatment, including palliative care of hyperkeratosis and functional orthotics to equilibrate ground reactive forces against the foot, will suffice. Surgical treatment to correct an intrinsic rearfoot varus (i.e., Dwyer osteotomy) is usually reserved for severe cases associated with chronic ankle sprains.

Partially Compensated Rearfoot Varus

In partially compensated rearfoot varus, the rearfoot partially pronates, but not enough to get the forefoot to the ground, causing increased motion in the forefoot, especially at the lateral aspect. Excess motion at the fifth ray leads to a tailor's bunion. With the fifth metatarsal bowing laterally, the flexor digitorum longus tendon no longer pulls the fifth toe straight but allows it to curl inward. If the fifth ray is mobile enough, a submetatarsal four hyperkeratotic lesion may develop due to decreased weight bearing at the fifth metatarsal. Again, functional foot orthoses to equilibrate the ground forces and control pronation, along with palliative care, constitute the conservative treatment of choice. If the tailor's bunion becomes symptomatic and painful, surgery is indicated.

Fully Compensated Rearfoot Varus

In fully compensated rearfoot varus, the patient is able to pronate the STJ so that the forefoot is placed totally on the ground. However, rearfoot pronation can cause irritation of the posterior heel, leading to a "pump bump" or Haglund's deformity (see Chapter 9). In addition, metatarsus primus elevatus can develop due to ground reactive forces pushing up on the first ray after the rearfoot pronates to the perpendicular position. Because of constant pounding of the first ray during gait, a hallux limitus develops over time that leads to a dorsal bunion and pain.

Conservative treatment modalities include functional foot orthoses to eliminate excessive pronation. Haglund's deformity is treated according to the guidelines outlined in Chapter 9. If hallux limitus develops, surgical intervention to remove the dorsal bunion and correct the elevated first metatarsal is indicated. If it is noted that the first metatarsophalangeal joint articular cartilage has undergone significant degenerative changes, the joint will need to be resected (i.e., Keller bunionectomy) to eliminate the pain.

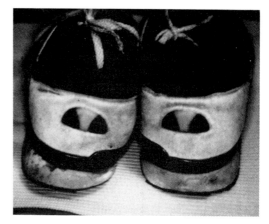

FIGURE 2. Medial heel wear of sneaker due to foot striking ground in valgus position.

Rearfoot Valgus

With a rearfoot valgus deformity, the foot strikes the ground everted (Fig. 2). This is caused by subtalar valgus, an intrinsic osseous abnormality in which the talus undergoes too much external rotation at birth, or by lower-extremity abnormalities such as genu valgus, a soft tissue or osseous abnormality at the knee joint causing the foot to maintain an everted relationship to the leg. In all cases, the heel strikes the ground beyond perpendicular (Fig. 3). A flatfoot type is usually observable (Fig. 4). Another cause of rearfoot valgus is a peroneal spastic flatfoot that is usually associated with tarsal coalition (i.e., fusion between tarsal bones) (see Chapter 10). When the patient tries to supinate the foot, pain is caused by the coalition. The peroneus brevis tries to hold the foot in an everted position to prevent pain, thus maintaining the flatfoot condition.

In forefoot supinatus associated with rearfoot valgus with the rearfoot hitting the ground everted, the medial column of the foot is unlocked. The ground pushes up on the medial column of the foot and maintains the forefoot in a supinated position. The supinated position is held in place by soft tissue that eventually adapts and maintains the supinated attitude. These patients walk with an awkward, clumsy gait. Once subtalar pronation is eliminated, the supinatus can be reversed.

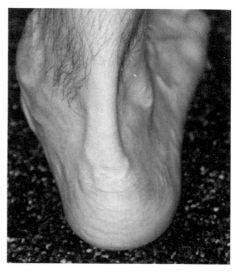

FIGURE 3. Valgus heel secondary to flatfoot.

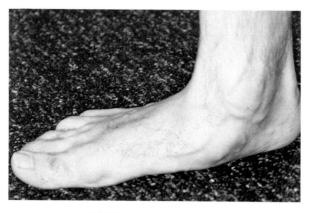

FIGURE 4. Severe flatfoot.

Nonsurgical treatment of rearfoot valgus includes orthotics that do not allow any motion at the subtalar joint, so that pain is prevented during ambulation. Conservative treatment of tarsal coalition also includes orthotics fabricated to prevent motion. Surgical intervention for the painful tarsal coalition in which conservative methods have failed includes a triple arthrodesis. The rearfoot valgus foot type is a very difficult foot to manage. The practitioner must deal with the foot symptomatically and try to provide comfort. Because the patient strikes the ground in a pronated position and thus unlocks the medial column, bunions are likely to develop; yet, if corrected surgically, they are likely to recur because excessive rearfoot pronation was not addressed.

OVERVIEW OF FOREFOOT VARUS AND VALGUS

At birth, the forefoot should be perpendicular to the rearfoot due to intrauterine external rotation of the talar neck. If this torsion does not take place, then forefoot varus, a one-plane osseous deformity, develops (see Chapter 10). Assessment is made by placing the STJ in neutral position, maximally pronating the midtarsal joint (MTJ) (loading the fifth metatarsal head via plantar pressure using the thumb), and noting the inverted relationship of the forefoot to the rearfoot. Forefoot valgus is also an osseous deformity in which the forefoot is everted relative to the rearfoot.

Forefoot Supinatus

Forefoot supinatus is a triplane soft tissue deformity caused by an inversion force applied to the forefoot during gait. If this force is maintained, the soft tissue adapts to this inverting force. Forefoot supinatus is generally caused by eversion of the rearfoot during gait.

Forefoot Varus

Metatarsals one through five are inverted relative to the rearfoot. In a forefoot varus deformity, which is an osseous abnormality of the talus, the talar neck does not undergo its full valgus torque at birth, thus allowing the metatarsals to become perpendicular to the rearfoot.

Clinically, the rearfoot hits the ground and undergoes a normal amount of eversion, yet in order to get the medial column of the forefoot down, the foot must pronate beyond rearfoot perpendicular. Once the STJ pronates to its maximum extent, other methods of compensation may or may not come into effect.

Uncompensated Forefoot Varus

In uncompensated forefoot varus, the first ray will plantarflex as in uncompensated rearfoot varus, but the calcaneus will be perpendicular to the ground (i.e., inverted with rearfoot varus). Calluses are observed under the first and fifth metatarsal heads.

Palliative care for the calluses immediately relieves discomfort under the first and fifth metatarsal heads, and functional foot orthoses aid in reducing and possibly eliminating the callus formation.

Partially Compensated Forefoot Varus

In partially compensated forefoot varus, the STJ and MTJ pronate, yet the MTJ does not pronate to allow full compensation. As in partially compensated rearfoot varus, a tailor's bunion, curled fifth digit, and hyperkeratosis submetatarsal four also develop because of a hypermobile fifth ray.

Functional foot orthoses fabricated with a forefoot post will, in essence, bring the ground up to the forefoot, thus eliminating the need for excessive pronation at the STJ and MTJ. Callus formation is palliatively treated through paring. If the tailor's bunion or curled fifth digit causes the patient severe pain, surgical intervention is indicated followed by functional foot orthoses to maintain correction.

Fully Compensated Forefoot Varus

Compensated forefoot varus occurs when the STJ everts beyond perpendicular. The midtarsal joint (MTJ) also compensates by pronating during midstance in an attempt to get the medial column down. The MTJ remains mobile during propulsion, causing the ground reactive forces to push the hallux into abduction during propulsion and resulting in a bunion deformity. If this bunion is not managed, lateral drifting of the hallux can result in increased pressure on the lateral aspect of the big toenail by the second toe, leading to an ingrown toenail. Continued hallux pressure can also cause the second digit to contract, resulting in a hammer toe or hallux overlap. Either of these situations will, in time, cause a subluxed second metatarsophalangeal joint (MPJ) and development of hyperkeratosis under the second metatarsal head.

In addition, heel spur syndrome (Chapter 9) can also occur with compensated forefoot varus. When the STJ and MPJ pronate, the arch of the foot drops, leading to pulling of the plantar fascia. When the fascia is torn away from the bone, bleeding develops and more bone is deposited, leading to the formation of a spur.

Functional foot orthoses fabricated in a manner similar to that for partially compensated forefoot varus constitute an excellent, conservative treatment of choice. If the fully compensated forefoot varus deformity is discovered after a painful bunion has developed, orthotics may slow the progress of the deformity but will not correct the bunion. Padding of the bunion as well as change of shoe gear (e.g., pumps changed to tennis shoes) can provide relief. Surgical correction of the bunion is reserved for intractable pain or cosmesis.

Forefoot Valgus

In a forefoot valgus deformity, the forefoot is everted relative to the rearfoot, and metatarsals one through five are everted relative to the calcaneus. This is a bony deformity in which valgus torsion during development of the talus is excessive. Sometimes the patient has a combination of forefoot valgus and rearfoot varus, resulting in a high arched or cavovarus foot type, a static deformity. If the patient notices in time that the arch is getting higher, the deformity is progressive. It would be prudent to look for neuromuscular problems creating this deformity such as Charcot-Marie-Tooth disease or Friedreich's ataxia.

If the patient is able to compensate for the forefoot valgus, pronation occurs at the MTJ or STJ. If the patient's ligaments are flexible, compensation occurs at the MTJ, and a flatfoot due to pronation results (flexible forefoot valgus). With this foot type, problems such as bunions, submetatarsal two calluses, hammer toes, or heel spur syndrome may develop.

If there is insufficient flexibility at the MTJ, compensation occurs at the STJ. The foot maintains the forefoot-to-rearfoot valgus relationship with weight bearing, and a rigid forefoot valgus develops. Problems associated with this foot include poor shock absorption resulting in back problems and "pump bump" or posterior heel irritation. Callus formation on submetatarsal one and five can appear along the plantar aspect of the foot. In time, the rearfoot may invert in an attempt to have the forefoot and rearfoot weight bearing during midstance. The chance of lateral ankle sprains increases proportionately.

Treatment options for flexible and rigid deformities include orthotics, primarily to support the deformity; palliative care for the calluses; surgical procedures to get the rearfoot out of varus; and dorsiflexory osteotomies of the metatarsals to get the forefoot out of valgus.

Surgical correction of a painful bunion and heel spurs followed by application of functional foot orthoses to maintain correction are reserved for severe, painful deformity.

HAMMER TOES

There are two types of hammer toes: static (or rigid) and dynamic. Static hammer toes are due to intrinsic osseous abnormalities. They account for 20% of all hammer toe deformities. Dynamic hammer toes are caused by intrinsic muscle fatigue. They account for 80% of all hammer toe deformities. There are three subtypes of dynamic hammer toes: extensor substitution, flexor stabilization, and flexor substitution.

Extensor substitution hammer toes occur when the long extensor muscles overpower the lumbricales. The lumbricales act to stabilize the digits during swing and counteract the extensor digitorum longus pull. When weakened, as occurs with a high-arched supinated foot, hammer toes develop.

Flexor stabilization hammer toes occur during the stance phase when the interossei muscles are overpowered by the flexor digitorum longus (FDL). When abnormal pronation occurs, the pull of the FDL is altered in the pronatory direction, causing an increased pull of the distal phalanx of toes two through five, in excess of the pull of the interossei.

Flexor substitution hammer toes are rare. They occur when the deep posterior leg muscles gain advantage over the intrinsic foot muscles due to weak superficial posterior leg muscles (the gastrocnemius-soleus complex).

If diagnosed early, the abnormal muscle forces of dynamic hammer toes can be corrected (without surgical intervention) via the use of functional foot orthoses in the cases of flexor stabilization and substitution hammer toes. Extensor substitution hammer toes almost always require surgical intervention. Generally, the patient has a painful hyperkeratosis over the proximal interphalangeal joint. At this stage, the dynamic hammer toe is rigid, and surgical intervention is usually required to correct the deformity. Sometimes the patient chooses to live with the deformity, in which case routine palliation consists of debridement; padding is the treatment of choice to provide the patient with relief from painful hammer toes.

BIBLIOGRAPHY

1. Jones JL, et al: Abnormal biomechanics of flatfoot deformities and related theories of biomechanical development. Clin Podiatr Med Surg 6:511–520, 1989.
2. Levitz SJ, et al: Biomechanical foot therapy. Clin Podiatr Med Surg 5:721–736, 1988.

Chapter 13

TRAUMA

Michael P. DellaCorte, D.P.M.,
Richard B. Birrer, M.D.,
and Paul V. Porcelli, D.P.M.

Injury to the foot and ankle from physical and recreational activities is remarkably common. Sports generate higher injury rates; industry produces more expensive and more serious injuries. The overall injury rate is 10–15 per 100 persons per year, most frequently involving the 17- to 44-year-old age group. Males are injured more often than females. The spectrum of injury comprises abrasions and lacerations (30%), sprains and strains (23%), contusions (20%), fractures and dislocations (10%), burns (3%), and miscellaneous trauma (e.g., electrical, chemical) (14%). Although most injuries are mild to moderate in nature, severe injury to the foot may occur in association with life-threatening trauma to the patient (e.g., a motor vehicle accident). Thus, if the patient is seen during the first 20–30 minutes following trauma (i.e., the so-called golden period), symptoms and signs are minimal to nonexistent. As time passes, symptoms, particularly pain, and signs, such as edema and discoloration, become more pronounced.

The management of the trauma patient begins with the ABCs of resuscitation (airway, breathing, and circulation) and continues with primary assessment and stabilization of life-threatening injuries (e.g., hemorrhage, sucking chest wounds, head injury). Failure to follow basic and advanced cardiac and trauma life support guidelines results in excessive morbidity and mortality. Focusing solely on pedal pathology without undressing the patient and considering nonpedal trauma may cause important associated injuries (e.g., entrance and exit wounds, vertebral fractures) to go unnoticed.

Once the patient is stabilized, a history of the injury should be obtained. Workers' compensation cases require an account of the injury in the patient's words. Useful questions include: What position was your foot in, relative to your body, when the injury occurred (i.e., inverted, everted, dorsiflexed, plantarflexed)? Did you hear or feel any snapping or cracking? Were you able to continue activities, or were you forced to stop because of the injury? What were you wearing on your feet at the time? (It is important to learn if shoes and socks were being worn and what type they were, because particles of these materials may have entered the wound during the injury if it was, for instance, a puncture wound.) Were you able to walk after the injury? Was there any treatment, and, if so, what were the results? Was the foot ever injured previously? The patient's medical and surgical history, including medications and allergies, should also be obtained and noted.

A detailed clinical examination of the foot follows. Too often lab tests and radiographs are ordered and interpreted as normal and the patient discharged without a thorough examination. The clinical evaluation should consist of inspection (e.g., for erythema, ecchymosis, edema, abrasions, and breaks in the skin), palpation (e.g., trigger points, range of motion, neurovascular status), and auscultation (osteophony).

INJURIES TO SKIN AND NAILS

Partial or complete nail avulsion can be caused by indirect or direct trauma (e.g., a lawn mower accident). In such cases, if examination of the nail bed shows it is badly lacerated, the first step is to repair it. Local anesthesia and a sterile suture tray are necessary. For the partially avulsed nail, there are two schools of thought on how to treat the injury. After x-rays have been taken and reveal no bone involvement, either the nail is completely avulsed or it is put back in place and bandaged. On one hand, complete nail avulsion may cause more trauma to an already injured area. On the other, leaving the nail on may allow the injured nail to act as a splint or guide for the new nail to follow. Some clinicians feel, however, that it may create a deformed new nail because it blocks growth. The authors recommend that the amount of trauma be assessed, and, if no anesthesia is necessary to avulse the nail completely, then avulsion should be performed. If it is more complicated than that, the nail should be soaked, and soaks prescribed. Reevaluation is made after two days; if the nail is stable, it should be left; if it is falling off, the patient should be followed until the nail falls off by itself.

Lacerations are tears in the skin from numerous causes. Learning the mechanism of injury is important since it will give the practitioner some idea as to whether he or she is dealing with a foreign body (e.g., glass, wood, stone) along with a laceration. Most glass is radiopaque, so x-ray evaluation may aid the treatment plan. Treatment of a laceration associated with a foreign body consists of local anesthesia, probing and removal of any foreign bodies, and flushing of the wound. Prior to suturing the laceration, a follow-up x-ray, to determine if all the foreign bodies have been removed, is advisable. Tetanus immunization status should be checked, and tetanus toxoid 0.5 ml given intramuscularly according to the guidelines in Table 1.

If the laceration does not involve any foreign bodies, it should be sutured primarily. Simple interrupted sutures with 4-0 nylon are recommended (see Chapter 20). They should remain clean and intact for 10–14 days. The wound should be examined 3, 7, and 14 days after injury, at which time they should be removed. If the laceration is on the plantar surface of the foot, the patient should not bear any weight for 2 weeks so as to reduce pressure on the wound and avoid gapping and suture disruption.

For a discussion of subungual hematoma, refer to Chapter 5.

TABLE 1. Guidelines for Antitetanus Treatment of Patients with Open Wounds

Tetanus Immunization History	Clean, Minor Wounds		All Other Wounds*	
	TD[†]	TIG	Td	TIG
Unknown or 0–2 doses	Yes	No	Yes	Yes
Three or more doses	No[‡]	No	No[§]	No

(Adapted from Tetanus—United States, 1987 and 1988, MMWR 39:37–41, Jan. 26, 1990.)

* Dirty wounds include contamination with dirt, feces, soil, or saliva; puncture wounds; avulsions; and wounds from missiles, crushing trauma, frostbite, or burns.

[†] Give diphtheria-pertussis-tetanus vaccine if less than 7 years old (or diphtheria-tetanus vaccine if pertussis is contraindicated).

[‡] If more than 10 years since last dose, give Td booster.

[§] If more than 5 years since last does, give Td booster.

(Td = Adult tetanus toxoid and diphtheria vaccine; TIG = tetanus immunoglobulin)

ANIMAL BITES

Most lower-extremity animal bites come from domestic animals and differ from human bites in that the wound contains fewer bacteria. Typical pathogens are *Staphylococcus aureus*, *Pasteurella multocida*, and anaerobes. Treatment consists of meticulous scrubbing with a bacteriostatic agent, thorough irrigation, debridement if needed, and closure. If the wound is large, contaminated, or a deep puncture, it should not be closed. Tetanus prophylaxis should be given according to the guidelines in Table 1. A broad-spectrum oral antibiotic such as cephalexin should be administered therapeutically (i.e., for a contaminated wound; an associated disease such as diabetes, peripheral vascular disease [PVD], or immunosupression; or presentation delayed for more than 8 hours), not prophylactically. Rabies vaccination is indicated in high-risk situations (e.g., bites by a raccoon, skunk, bat, fox, or unhealthy cat or dog that has escaped).

INJURIES TO SUBCUTANEOUS TISSUE

Puncture wounds to the plantar surface of the foot often appear innocuous but represent a diagnostic and therapeutic dilemma to the primary care physician. A total of 5.8% of lower-extremity trauma involves a puncture injury, with a seasonal variation favoring the warmer months. Nails are the most common

(98%), but other objects such as glass, metal, wood, and plastic can serve as a wounding agent. Depth of penetration seems to be the most critical factor affecting outcome, although elapsed time to presentation is also a predictor of potential poor outcome. Overall, puncture wounds have a low incidence of complications, but both difficulty in judging depth of penetration and the potential presence of retained foreign bodies place these wounds at a high risk. The infection rate appears to be less than 3% and the incidence of osteomyelitis less than 1%. A careful history (e.g., type of footwear and puncture object) and examination of the wound are indicated for injuries of less than 24 hours. Epidermal flaps should be trimmed, the wound cleansed, and the tetanus vaccination updated if indicated (see Table 1). Irrigation may be counterproductive; probing requires a regional nerve block and has an unknown false-negative rate. Coring using a cuticle scissors, No. 11 scalpel blade, or 4-mm punch biopsy enhances drainage and visualization. Soft tissue radiography, computerized tomography (CT), magnetic resonance imaging (MRI), or ultrasound should be performed whenever there is a question of the possibility of a retained foreign body. Very superficial foreign bodies can be soaked for a few days and then removed in the office with minimal anesthesia. The anesthesia should be placed proximal to the foreign body. If the injection is too close to the portal of entry, it may distort tissue architecture and float the foreign body. Deeper foreign bodies should be handled in the operating room, where the object can be triangulated by fluoroscopy (mini C arm) and surgically excised. Puncture wounds without lacerations should not be closed but, rather, allowed to granulate. Antibiotics (i.e., broad-spectrum antistaphylococcal antibiotics such as cephalexin) for 7–10 days are generally reserved for high-risk wounds (e.g., in the compromised patient with diabetes or PVD after 24 hours and in patients who present with signs of local infection, a draining tract, a grossly contaminated wound, or a foreign object that may have penetrated to bone joint space or plantar fascia). The suspicion of a deep space infection, the failure of a cellulitis to respond to antibiotics, a relapse, or a draining tract should suggest an osteomyelitis. More than 90% of such cases are caused by a *Pseudomonas* species. A bone scan should be obtained rapidly because in the early stages, it is much more sensitive than a radiograph.

TABLE 2.   *Common Sites of Bursitis*

Medial first metatarsophalangeal joint
Lateral fifth metatarsophalangeal joint
Lateral fifth metatarsal base
Dorsal interphalangeal joints of the toes
Navicular tuberosity
Plantar aspect—metatarsal head
Posterior to the calcaneus (see Chapter 9)

BURSITIS

A bursa is a sac or a saclike cavity that is filled with a viscous fluid and is located at a frictional site in the tissues. An adventitial bursa is an abnormal bursa. Bursitis due to acute trauma or overuse is often found at the joints of the foot that are exposed to pressure from a shoe. The most common sites are listed in Table 2.

A highly inflamed bursa must be differentiated from infection, joint effusion, and arthritic conditions. On examination, the area will usually be elevated and circumscribed. Its surface can range from smooth and soft to firm with hyperkeratotic tissue. Acute bursitis will be tender to palpation and movement of the area, as well as erythematous and edematous with an associated temperature increase.

Treatment of acute bursitis includes elimination of the trauma and protection of the area from future irritation; aspiration; ice therapy; nonsteroidal anti-inflammatory drugs (NSAIDs); Burow's solution soaks; and injection therapy to relieve swelling and acute pain. Antibiotics are prescribed if a secondary infection is present. In chronic bursitis, surgical excision of the bursa and the underlying bone is often necessary. A consultation is warranted.

CONTUSION

A contusion is an injury to the soft tissue from a direct or indirect blow without disruption of the skin. Edema, erythema, ecchymosis, and temperature increase of the area are usually present. Pain may be associated with palpation and occasionally with range of motion. X-ray evaluation must be performed in order to rule out osseous pathology.

Treatment consists of rest, ice, compression, and elevation (RICE), horseshoe padding, NSAIDs, analgesics, and possible nonweight-bearing of the affected foot. Physical therapy should be started after the acute inflammation has subsided in order to reduce edema and increase pain-free range of motion and strength.

DISLOCATION

Pure dislocation is rare in the foot. The metatarsophalangeal joints are the most common joints involved in a pure dislocation. The proximal phalanx is displaced upward and backward in the vertical position. The distal phalanx is flexed. X-ray evaluation confirms the diagnosis. The lateral view reveals the proximal phalanx resting on the metatarsal head; the dorsal plantar shows the same with a gun barrel sign of the proximal phalanx. Immediate reduction is mandatory.

Local anesthesia is administered proximal to the metatarsophalangeal joint on both sides of the involved metatarsal. After the area is blocked, a gauze pad is applied around the involved digit. Gripping the gauze pad and the toe firmly, the examiner pulls the toe upward and proximal; continuing the upward pull, the examiner then brings the toe distally (forward) and downward, back in place. Bone-to-bone contact should not be felt, indicating that the upward distraction was not sufficient. Bone rubbing can cause fractures and more trauma. A splint should be applied to the foot to prevent recurrent hyperextension of the involved joint. Crutch walking for 2–3 weeks to prevent the toe-off stage of gait and further dislocation may be necessary. Physical therapy and a postsurgical shoe should be worn until symptoms resolve.

TRAUMA TO BONE: FOOT FRACTURES

Digital Fractures

Digital fractures are generally caused by direct trauma to the involved toe (Fig. 1). Left untreated, these fractures can result in painful bony prominences and helomas. The most commonly fractured toe is the fifth toe. Stubbing the toe in bare or stocking feet is the usual cause. Clinically, the digit is ecchymotic, edematous, warm, and painful. Anteroposterior and lateral films demonstrate the fracture, although comparison x-rays may be necessary.

Treatment is determined by the degree or severity of the fracture and associated injury. A simple nondisplaced digital fracture of the

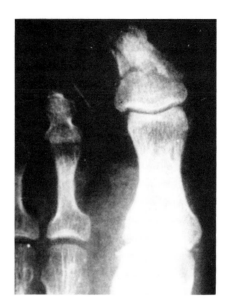

FIGURE 1.   Digital fracture of hallux–distal phalanx.

lesser digits can be treated by buddy splinting the fractured digit to the neighboring uninjured digit. A piece of gauze or cotton is placed between the toes being splinted, and half-inch tape is basket-weaved around the digits. It is important never to circumscribe the digits, since the tape would act as a tourniquet around the toes and cut off circulation if there is further swelling. The basket weave, on the other hand, allows for expansion. Early ambulation in a protective shoe allows the majority of toe fractures to heal in 4–5 weeks. Amputation, however, may be necessary for fractures associated with severe crush injuries. Careful follow-up is essential, because a moderate degree of angulation or rotation of the toes can produce functional disability. Posttraumatic arthritis and hammer-toe deformity are perhaps the most significant disabilities possible and are best prevented by avoiding reinjury as well as carefully rehabilitating the injured foot in a progressive fashion.

Sesamoidal Fractures

The two sesamoids in the flexor hallucis brevis tendon can be fractured by direct trauma or hyperextension of the hallux. The tibial sesamoid is fractured more often than the fibular (Fig. 2). Symptoms include pain, particularly when stair climbing and wearing high-heel shoes. There may be minimal to significant edema, trigger point tenderness,

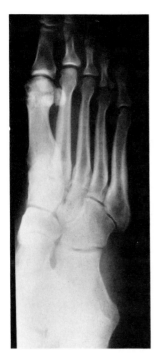

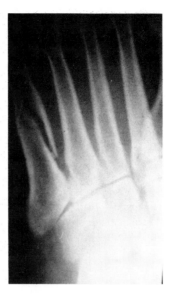

FIGURE 3. Fracture of fifth metatarsal.

FIGURE 2. Fracture of the tibial sesamoid and proximal second phalanx following a crush injury.

and tenderness and ecchymosis of the metatarsophalangeal joint.

Treatment is determined by degree of injury. Nondisplaced fractures are treated with dispersion padding and low-heel shoes. Off-weightbearing and short-leg-cast immobilization may be necessary if symptoms do not subside. Displaced fractures should be cast and remain nonweightbearing for 4–6 weeks. If left untreated, sesamoid fractures may progress to painful nonunion. Surgical excision should be considered.

Metatarsal Fractures

Metatarsal fractures (Figs. 3 to 6) may result from direct or indirect trauma. The site of the fracture (i.e., the epiphysis, metaphysis, diaphysis, or intra-articular) is important. The metaphyseal area has the best blood supply and therefore will heal the quickest, whereas the diaphysis and epiphysis have decreased vascularity, requiring longer immobilization. The diagnosis and degree of injury are determined by patient history, physical exam, and x-ray. Dorsal plantar (DP), lateral, and oblique radiographic views are advised. The DP x-ray

shows transverse plane deviation; the lateral demonstrates sagittal plane deviation. The five metatarsals are viewed as internal (2, 3, and 4), and external (1 and 5). The external metatarsals have a greater biomechanical demand (i.e., weightbearing) and generally need almost perfect alignment and rigid fixation. The fifth metatarsal is subject to two types of fractures at the base. The first is an avulsion fracture of the base caused by the peroneus brevis during inversion sprains. The second is the Jones fracture, which is a transverse, usually nondisplaced fracture of the proximal diaphyseal area.

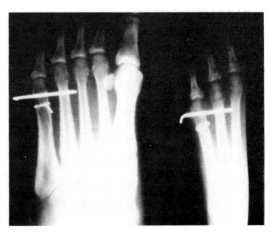

FIGURE 4. Open reduction with internal fixation of fracture in Figure 3.

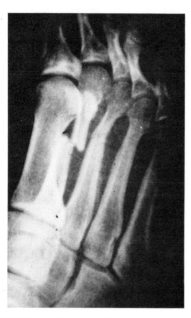

FIGURE 5. Fracture of second metatarsal.

Treatment should be geared to the age and physical condition of the patient. For a nondisplaced fracture without associated crush injury, a short-leg cast is indicated for 4–6 weeks. The Unna boot and Ace bandage along with a shoe with a rigid shank or sole (Reece) for 4–6 weeks can be used on patients who cannot tolerate a cast. Dorsally or plantarly displaced, angulated, or multiple metatarsal fractures, fracture dislocations, or extensive crush injuries with no bone-to-bone contact and gapping greater than 4 mm should be treated in the operating room for open reduction and internal fixation, if closed reduction fails. Fasciotomy, along with other soft tissue releases, may be required to reduce the fracture. Hospitalization and close observation are essential. If these fractures are not fixated and the patient is allowed to ambulate in a soft cast (Unna boot), the unstable distal metatarsal will become dorsally displaced. Once healed in this position, it will bear minimal weight, subjecting the patient to possible plantar helomas under the other metatarsals now bearing more weight.

Avulsion fractures to the fifth metatarsal, if nondisplaced, generally respond well to a soft cast and postoperative shoe used for 4–6 weeks. If there is displacement, closed reduction, and nonweightbearing, a short-leg cast should be used. Open reduction and internal fixation may be necessary if closed reduction fails; a specialist should be consulted. Jones fractures of the fifth metatarsal base have a very high incidence of pseudarthrosis due to the location of the fracture and poor blood supply. Therefore, these fractures require off-weight short-leg casts for 6–8 weeks if closed reduction is successful. Surgical intervention is necessary when closed reduction fails or when there is either delayed union or nonunion.

Cuneiform Fractures

These fractures follow direct trauma and are usually associated with other fractures, injuries, or both. The medial cuneiform is the most likely to be affected. Treatment consists of compression dressing or casting, depending on the severity of the fracture. A specialist should be consulted.

Navicular Fractures

Watson Jones classified navicular fractures into three categories: type I, fracture of the tuberosity; type II, fracture of the dorsal lip; and type III, transverse body fracture. These fractures can be caused by forceful eversion of the foot or direct trauma. It is important to distinguish tuberosity fractures from the presence of an os tibiale externum, which is an

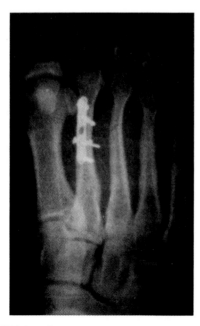

FIGURE 6. Open reduction with internal fixation of fracture in Figure 5.

accessory bone on the medial aspect on the navicular. Comparison x-rays are indicated, since the accessory bone will be present bilaterally. Treatment consists of a non-weight-bearing short-leg cast for 4–6 weeks, depending on the severity of the injury. Open reduction with internal fixation may be indicated. Foot orthotics may be needed after immobilization.

Cuboid Fractures

This is an uncommon fracture, usually resulting from compression forces or direct trauma (Fig 7). Conservative treatment consists of cast immobilization for 4–6 weeks. A specialist should be consulted.

Talar Fractures

Although the primary care physician will probably not treat talar fractures, recognition is necessary before a specialist is consulted. The most common fractures involve the dome, neck, or body, although combination injuries (fractures, dislocations) are not uncommon. Talar fractures are usually associated with ankle injuries.

Talar Dome Fractures

Berndt-Harty has classified talar dome fractures into four stages: I, subchondral bone compression; II, partially detached fragment; III, completely detached nondisplaced fragment; and IV, completely detached displaced fragment. The mechanism of injury is inversion. The patient presents an ankle sprain that does not respond to conservative treatment. Dome fractures are difficult to visualize on standard x-ray views; a CT scan or MRI is needed for definitive diagnosis. Treatment may involve casting, arthroscopy, and/or surgical excision of any loose fragments. A specialist should be consulted.

Talar Neck Fractures

Talar neck fractures can be caused by car accidents, falls from heights, direct trauma from falling objects, or athletic injuries.

The Hawkins classification for talar neck fractures is as follows: type I, vertical fracture through the talar neck without displacement of the talar body; type II, vertical fracture through

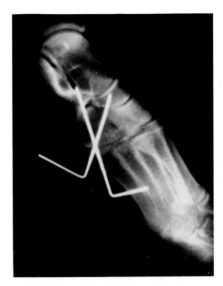

FIGURE 7. Cuboid fracture fixated with cross "K" wires.

the neck with subtalar joint subluxation or dislocation; type III, vertical fracture of talar neck with displacement of the talar body from the subtalar and tibiotalar joints; and type IV, vertical fracture of the talar neck with talar body displacement from both subtalar and tibiotalar joints and subluxation and/or dislocation of the talar head from the talonavicular joint.

The probability of avascular necrosis of the talus increases greatly from type I to type IV. Treatment ranges from casting to open reduction, depending on the degree of fracture. The average length of casting is 8–14 weeks. A specialist should be consulted.

Talar Body

Talar body fractures are not as common as talar neck fractures, and the prognosis is not as good. A small amount of incongruity caused by the injury may cause a step deformity and subsequent posttraumatic arthritis. Anatomic reduction should be attempted by a specialist, but even with good reduction, a painless joint may never be restored. Initial treatment ranges from casting to open reduction. Long-term management may require joint fusion.

Calcaneal Fractures

Calcaneal fractures (Fig. 8) are the most common of all tarsal fractures, with an incidence of approximately 60%. The thin outer

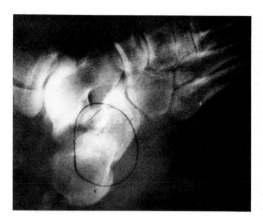

FIGURE 8.   Calcaneal fracture.

cortical shell and soft cancellous bone of the calcaneus make it easily susceptible to traumatic injuries. The majority of fractures are caused by falls from a height. For instance, rapid egress from an upper-floor window with a subsequent fall and os calcis fracture has been termed "lover's heel." Calcaneal fractures have a high incidence of associated injuries involving the spine, femur, fibula, tibia, talus, ulna, and radius.

These fractures have been classified into several different systems, making them easier to understand. Rowe classification of calcaneal fractures is as follows: type I (A) fractures of the tuberosity, (B) fractures of the sustentaculum tali, and (C) fractures of the anterior process; type II (A) beak fractures and (B) avulsion fractures of the Achilles tendon insertion; type III, oblique fractures not involving the subtalar joint; type IV, fractures involving the subtalar joint; and type V, central depression fractures with varying degrees of comminution.

The complex nature and prognosis of calcaneal fractures require the expertise of a specialist.

ANKLE FRACTURES

The mechanism of injury and the structures involved in ankle fractures have been classified by Lauge-Hansen. There are two terms that describe the injury. The first term describes the position of the foot at the time of injury; the second refers to the direction of the pathologic forces being applied to the talus (the position of the leg).

Supination adduction trauma causes either a transverse avulsion fracture of the fibula at or below the ankle joint or a rupture of the lateral collateral ligaments (stage I). If the pathologic force continues, an oblique-to-vertical fracture of the medial malleolus occurs (stage II). Supination eversion (external rotation) injuries begin with rupture of the anterior inferior tibiofibular ligament (stage I). As the pathologic force continues, there is a spiral oblique fracture of the fibula beginning at the ankle joint (stage II) (Fig. 9), posterior inferior tibiofibular ligament rupture or posterior malleolar fracture (stage III), and finally medial malleolar fracture or deltoid ligament rupture (stage IV).

Pronation abduction trauma causes either a transverse fracture of the medial malleolus or a rupture of the deltoid ligament (stage I). If the pathologic force continues, a rupture of the anterior and posterior inferior tibiofibular ligaments will occur, or there will be avulsion fractures at the ligamentous attachment of the anterior and posterior inferior tibiofibular ligaments (stage II). Further progression to stage III causes a short, oblique fracture to the fibula. Pronation eversion (external rotation) injuries begin at the medial malleolus; as the pathologic force continues, the injury progresses as follows: transverse avulsion fracture of the medial malleolus or rupture of the deltoid ligaments (stage I), rupture of the anterior inferior tibiofibular ligament and interosseous membrane (stage II), high spiral

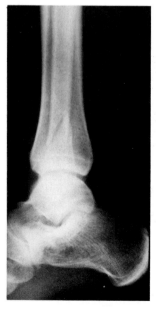

FIGURE 9.   Spiral fracture of the distal fibula associated with a deltoid ligament tear.

oblique fracture of the fibular (proximal extent of fracture depends on how high the interosseous ligament is ruptured) (stage III), and rupture of the posterior inferior tibiofibular ligament or avulsion fracture of the posterior malleolus (stage IV).

Stable injuries consist of one break in the mortise ring; unstable injuries consist of two or more breaks that may comprise any combination of fractures and ligament injuries. Symptoms include an audible pop or crack, abrupt moderate to severe pain and swelling, immediate disability, and delayed discoloration. Clinical signs consist of localized-point tenderness, edema, positive osteophony and tuning fork tests, possible crepitus, and ecchymosis. Associated trauma (i.e., ligamentous injury) should be suspected and diligently searched for. Results of the clinical evaluation may be very similar to those associated with a sprain of the ankle. Anteroposterior, lateral, and mortise views usually suffice to make the diagnosis. Stable injuries resulting from a single fracture or ligament tear require no reduction and can be treated with a posterior splint and the RICE regimen followed by a walking cast for 4–6 weeks. Unstable injuries due to a sprain, a fracture, or various combinations thereof require reduction. A specialist should be consulted. Initially closed manipulation, with or without local or general anesthesia, and muscle relaxants may be successful; however, open reduction is often required. Closed reduction is performed in three steps: exaggeration of the mechanism of injury, traction, and reversal of the mechanism of injury. A postreduction radiograph is essential. The medial portion of a fibular fracture at the syndesmosis unites rapidly, though the lateral half is slower or often does not heal at all due to the interposition of a narrow strip of periosteum from the proximal fragment's falling into the fracture line. Similarly, small avulsion fragments from the tip of the lateral malleolus or laterally angulated communicated fracture chips often do not reunite but serve as a source of localized osteoarthritis. Small distal fragments of the medial malleolus tend to be less easily reduced and are a source of frequent nonunion. Fractures of the lateral tibial margin (i.e., Tillaux fractures) are a frequent source of nonunion or malunion. Posterior tibial margin fractures usually heal well, with a return of good function. One exception involves fracture of more than one third of the tibial articular surface, in which the displaced surface of the talus and tibia results in damage to the articular surface of the mortise. Despite good reduction, osteoarthritis is a frequent sequela. Compression fractures often lead to degenerative joint disease due to the profound amount of damage to the involved articular surfaces, disruption of blood supply, and most commonly associated infections if the fracture is open. Therefore, ongoing clinical evaluation, including radiographs in conjunction with a consultant for unstable fractures, is essential.

Isometric exercises and a plaster cast or early range-of-motion exercises in a hinge cast will minimize the harmful effects of immobilization (e.g., stiffness and muscle atrophy). Internal fixation devices should generally be removed before the athlete is allowed to return to play in contact sports. Unstable injuries tend to have a very high incidence of complication (e.g., traumatic arthritis, persistent talar instability, Sudeck's atrophy, or ossification of the interosseous membrane).

Small fragments of subchondral bone and overlying articular cartilage can be separated from the talar dome due to compression or repetitive shearing-type loads, particularly in forced plantar flexion (i.e., a missed jump). The lesion may be located anywhere on the talar dome but commonly involves the superomedial and lateral margins. Such injuries tend to be unilateral and often are associated with old sprains, although the cause-and-effect relationship has not been definitively established. There is a gradual onset of pain, which becomes worse over weeks and even months, intensifies with exercise, and usually causes ankle stiffness or locking. The clinical exam is, for the most part, unremarkable, except that palpation of the talar dome with the ankle in plantar flexion will elicit point tenderness. Although special radiographic views may visualize the lesion, radioisotope studies or CT scan will produce the best results. Osteonecrotic fragments tend to be unilateral, whereas osteochondritis dissecans tends to be bilateral. Arthroscopy and arthrography are also useful. Consultation should be considered, since the incidence of disabling traumatic arthritis is high.

Stress Fractures

Repetitive microtrauma from running can lead to a stress fracture of the distal fibula. Lateral ankle pain may suggest peroneal tendinitis or a sprain, but the onset of localized firm swelling should suggest the diagnosis.

Rest, with a slowly progressive training program within the limits of pain, is the treatment of choice.

Tenderness and soft tissue swelling about the distal fibular epiphysis following trauma must be considered a type I Salter-Harris fracture in a youngster. Although radiographs may be normal, immobilization in a short-leg cast for 4–5 weeks is appropriate.

Metatarsal Stress Fractures

A stress fracture, also known as march fracture or Deutschlander's disease, is an overuse injury. The history is notable for a change in distance, technique, training, or footwear and the absence of a traumatic event. Mild, dull pain occurs, gradually increases, and becomes incapacitating with continued activity. The foot becomes edematous and erythematous. Direct palpation causes severe localized pain. X-ray evaluation in the early stages is negative. X-rays should be repeated in 10–12 days. Radiographic findings may range from callus formation around the fracture to a complete break in the cortex. If repeat films are negative and stress fracture is suspected, a bone scan is indicated. The bone scan will be "hot" in the area of the fracture. Treatment consists of NSAIDs, analgesics as needed, and a soft cast (Unna boot) or a Jones compression bandage for 4–6 weeks. Off-weightbearing with crutches may be necessary if a postoperative shoe cannot be tolerated.

COMBINATION INJURIES

The potential for multiple injuries involving ligament, tendon, bone, and subcutaneous tissue cannot be overstressed in the trauma patient. Heightened vigilance will permit detection of ligamentous injury with an unstable mortise or an avulsion fracture following a sprain. Such injuries should be managed in conjunction with a specialist. Tetanus immunization and antibiotics should be initiated if the clinical situation warrants.

ENVIRONMENTAL INJURIES

Burns

Collectively, the feet and the ankle represent 10% of the body surface area. Because the feet are critical to all ambulatory activities, a burn can produce a disproportionate amount of disability. For one reason or other, burns of the feet are often overlooked and minimally rehabilitated. Industrially, the result is a significant degree of lost wages and productivity.

Burns can occur from a variety of agents: chemical, electrical, radiation, and thermal sources. The extent of the injury is determined primarily by the intensity and duration of contact. Less important factors, but nonetheless contributory to the overall degree of burns, include the patient's age and health status, as well as environmental factors such as protective gear. In etiology, though, the details of the treatment plan depend on the type of injury agent.

Etiology.   Common causes of thermal burns include scalding, contact with a heat source, and fire. The individual with PVD due to atherosclerosis or neuropathy in association with diabetes can easily suffer contact burns from a hot-water bottle due to impaired sensation. A common childhood accident is scalding by hot water, though the possibility of child abuse should always be considered in any child who has suffered a symmetrical burn with a distinct line of demarcation, as from immersion.

The foot is often involved in electrical burns. It serves as a site for entrance or exit of the current (e.g., high-voltage lines, lightning strikes). The amount of injury is determined by the voltage (low vs. high tension), amperage, current type (alternating current [AC] vs. direct current [DC]), area of the body through which the current passes, duration, resistance of body tissue structures, and environmental factors such as water and rubber insulation. More damage occurs following contact with an AC current due to tetanic muscle contractions, which cause localized necrosis, and the victim's holding onto the current source. The electric current may enter through the feet, pass through the trunk, and exit through the head, digits, or upper extremity, or vice versa. A zone of gray-white necrosis surrounding a central area of charring characterizes the entry site. A more peripheral circumferential zone is hyperemic and ischemic. The exit sites there may have no apparent clinical signs, although there is often extensive underlying soft tissue and organ damage. There may also be thrombosis of vessels, rupture of muscles, and fracture of bones. In diminishing order of resistance, the differing levels of resistance for each of the body tissues are skin, bone, fat, tendon, muscle, blood vessel, and nerve. The thickness of the skin enhances or detracts from resistance. With increasing amounts of resistance, greater amounts of thermal injury are induced.

Chemical injuries to the foot occur by a number of pathogenic mechanisms. Depending on the agent, there may be coagulation or liquefaction by oxidation, salt formation, corrosion, reduction, metabolic competitive inhibition, desiccation, or protoplasmic poisoning. These reactions may be accompanied by a variable degree of thermal activity. The type and amount of the agent, duration of contact, and local conditions determine the severity of the injury.

Lastly, radiation causes burns through its damage to cells by ionization. The amount of damage is related to the type of radiation (alpha, beta, or gamma particles, with the latter being the most penetrating) and the amount and duration of exposure. Acutely, death is usually due to the systemic effect of bone marrow suppression and gastrointestinal toxicity. Prolonged exposure over many years, in this case to the foot, causes a number of pathologic changes, including fibrotic scarring, endarteritis obliterans, and chromosomal changes at the cellular level. The most feared development is that of neoplasia. For this reason, a full-thickness skin biopsy should be performed on suspicious lesions following radiation injury.

Treatment. The management of acute burns begins with stabilization of the patient—the basic ABCs of resuscitation (airway, breathing, and circulation). The type of agent, time of occurrence, and a detailed description of how the burn occurred are then determined. A rough estimate of the amount of body surface burned should be made as should the depth and extent of the burn. It is difficult to assess burn depth accurately. The old classification system of first-, second-, and third-degree burns is more usefully replaced by partial- and full-thickness classifications. There is no simple method to determine whether the depth is partial or full, since such injuries are dynamically progressive. Careful inspection and testing for sensation by pinprick provide reasonably accurate information. The anesthetic, waxy appearance of skin that has a denuded epidermis is highly suggestive of a full-thickness burn. An erythematous area responsive to pinprick is considered a partial-thickness injury that can produce enough edema around the eschar to result in circulatory embarrassment.

With the exception of first-degree, partial-thickness injury, all patients who sustain burns of the feet should be admitted to the hospital. Escharotomy is often necessary, and the dependent nature of the foot predisposes it to poor healing, infection, and circulatory compromise. The burn should be evaluated, analgesics and adequate fluids provided, tetanus prophylaxis administered according to the hospital's burn protocol, and diligent wound care begun. Cooling of the burned area with water of approximately 77°F (25°C) for 30–45 minutes is probably the safest cooling method.

Very cold water, ice, and systemic hypothermia should be avoided because the depth and extent of necrosis may increase. Drying of the wound should also be avoided. Vesicles should be left intact; if tense, they can be aspirated, with the overlying epidermis left in place. Debridement of less necrotic tissue is acceptable, but excessive tissue removal should be avoided. A protective covering of hydroactive gel, petrolatum, or antiseptic ointment (e.g., DuoDerm, Xeroform) can be used on a superficial, partial-thickness injury. Deep partial thickness or full-thickness wounds must be protected from bacterial contamination due to the overlying necrosis. Such wounds should be handled in consultation with a surgeon. Grafting may be done immediately following an escharotomy, or it may be delayed. The use of antibiotic therapy depends on the severity of the burn, the overall health status of the patient, and the presence of complications (e.g., inhalation injury).

Neither topical nor systemic antibiotic therapy in burn wound management is obligatory. Usually one of the topical antibiotics—silver nitrate, mafenide acetate (Sulfamylon), or silver sulfadiazine (Silvadene)—is used, although none of the three is more efficacious than the other. Each of the agents is bacteriostatic. Up to 7% of patients are hypersensitive to mafenide acetate; it is also painful on administration. Silver sulfadiazine has been known to produce neutropenia in a small number of hypersensitive individuals. Silver nitrate can cause methemoglobinemia and, of course, a profound amount of staining. Most important, serial local and systemic cultures should be taken in order to determine the type and significance of secondary infection in the burn patient.

Finally, total management of the burn patient consists of adequate and early rehabilitation in order to prevent contracture formation.

Because most burns occur on the dorsum of the foot, contractures usually result in hyperextension and dorsiflexion of the metatarsophalangeal joints. Less commonly, plantar surface burns can cause deformities of the foot and toes in equinus and flexion. Such contractures follow deep partial-thickness and full-thickness burns or full-thickness burns to which autografts have been applied. Rehabilitation, when properly performed, begins during the initial care of the burn wound with the construction and application of a splint that will help prevent equinus deformity. Thereafter, a molded shoe with sufficient padding to oppose the contractile forces of the wound must be constructed in order to reduce scarring and fibrosis. A carefully tailored exercise program involving passive and active range of motion is essential. Surgical reconstruction is reserved for burns that have not responded to or that follow incomplete rehabilitation.

Brief mention should be made of the treatment for electrical burns. During the acute stage, immediate escharotomy and decompressive fasciotomy are essential, particularly for high-tension injuries. These are the best methods for controlling ischemia in the electrically injured foot. Thereafter, when the patient's condition has been stabilized, careful debridement of all necrotic tissue should be performed cautiously, as the full extent of the damage may become evident only over several days, particularly in the case of nerve injury.

With few exceptions (e.g., sodium metal), the application of liberal amounts of water is the best and most effective treatment for burns from chemical substances. The use of neutralizing agents, such as a weak base for an acid or vice versa, is not condoned because an exothermic reaction may result, causing further damage.

Cold Injuries

As with burns, the severity and extent of tissue damage to the foot by cold temperature are proportional to the duration of exposure, the ambient temperature and humidity, the presence of environmental factors such as stockings and footwear, the overall health and activity level of the individual (e.g., Raynaud's disease or phenomenon, PVD, and the amount of drug use (e.g., alcohol or nicotine). Limited cold exposure can cause acute frostbite of the forefoot. The indigent alcoholic

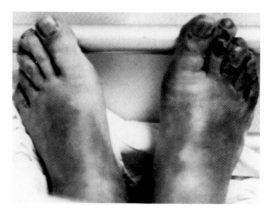

FIGURE 10. Necrosis and gangrene of toes following an alcoholic stupor in a snowdrift.

and elderly, particularly in the inner city, are most at risk. The patient complains of paresthesias and a cold, numb foot with waxy skin that becomes tingling and throbbing when warmed. Treatment consists of slow, progressive thawing by passive measures such as blankets and covers of warm water 40–42°C (100–104°F). Late sequelae of frostbite include vasomotor instability in mild cases (e.g., hyperhidrosis, paresthesias), necrosis, loss of digits, and contracture formation in severe frostbite (Fig. 10).

Related conditions include chilblains (pernio), trench foot, and immersion foot. The latter conditions were described during the two world wars, although they can be seen among outdoor enthusiasts (e.g., hunters and boaters). Freezing temperatures are not required in any of these conditions. Pathophysiologically, there is chronic injury to the sympathetic nerves and the microcirculation. Trench foot usually occurs during limited activity in a confined space such as a foxhole in cold, damp weather. After several days there is usually blanching of the foot, dusky cyanosis, superficial blister formation, and pain. With longer degrees of exposure, there is loss of the range of motion of the toes, diminution of sensation, and possible formation of gangrene. Immersion of the foot allows prolonged exposure to a cold, wet environment. Necrosis and maceration of the skin of the foot and leg are more significant than those seen in trench foot. Sequelae are similar though usually more severe. Treatment is supportive, with conservative debridement, control of infections, rest, elevation, early rehabilitation, and prevention of further exposure.

INDUSTRIAL AND OCCUPATIONAL FOOT INJURIES

Numerous reports have estimated that 9–16% of occupational injuries involve the foot and ankle. The amount of compensation for lost work productivity exceeds $1.2 billion each year. The majority of these injuries occur in workers doing heavy labor (49%), with the next largest single group being carpenters, who compose about 10% of the total. According to a recent Canadian Injury Survey of Foot and Ankle Injuries, the distribution was as follows: ankle (32%), heel (6%), sole (6%), toes (25%), and metatarsal region (31%). The majority of such injuries occur in young, inexperienced workers; males sustain injuries six times more frequently than females. The type of injury is equally distributed between the genders. Twenty-five to 30% of these injuries are secondary to slips or falls, particularly while the worker was hurrying. According to a number of surveys over the past 20 years, the incidence of foot and ankle industrial injuries is about 10%.

Recovery from a workers' compensation injury is often prolonged due to a number of factors. Psychologically it is difficult to resume a regular work schedule following a prolonged absence. In addition, there is usually increased pain upon the return to work. Moreover, the patient, through lack of understanding, often equates increased pain with increased damage and, therefore, the possibility of permanent injury. Finally, compensation payments are often equal to or may exceed after-tax income from the regular employment salary.

Regional Injuries

Toe. The majority of toe injuries occur from objects that fall on the foot. The spectrum of trauma ranges from minor soft tissue contusions to severe crush injury of the phalanges. The distal phalanx of the first toe has the highest incidence of fracture injury, followed by the first metatarsal. Combined, these two areas represent 50% of fractures. The fifth metatarsal is fractured 25% of the time, and the middle three metatarsal rays the remaining 25% of the time. The metatarsals may also be injured during forced plantar flexion; inversion through direct trauma, as from a blow, constitutes the most common etiology. Severe injuries are rare and include fracture dislocation at the tarsometatarsal joint (Lisfranc's fracture), fracture dislocation through the mid-tarsal joint (Chopart's fracture), and anterior crush injury. Most commonly there is soft tissue contusion, hemorrhage into the extensor digitorum brevis, and traumatic synovitis of the dorsal tendon sheaths.

Heel. Injuries to the heel are relatively uncommon in the industrial setting. The most common etiologies consist of a fall (e.g., among fire fighters and structural steel workers) or repetitive microtrauma (e.g., among military and marching band personnel) from hard, nonresilient surfaces during ambulation. The majority of such injuries usually involve contusions and possibly bursitis in the heel pad, which can result in chronic fibrotic scarring and can be a source of continued pain. Such injuries need to be distinguished from the plantar fasciitis derived from the anterior border of the calcaneal tuberosity, which can also result from industrial injury principally due to poorly fitting footwear and prolonged periods of standing, ambulation, or both (see Chapter 9). Calcaneal fractures have a poor prognosis regardless of treatment methodology. An orthopedic surgeon or podiatric surgeon should be consulted.

Plantar Region. Under ideal conditions in the industrial setting, injuries to the sole of the foot are relatively uncommon because of the use of safety boots with rigid steel shanks. Before the practice was required, the incidence of puncture wounds was often as high as 30–40% of all foot injuries among construction laborers. It has now fallen to 5–8%. Unlike puncture wounds, deep plantar lacerations rarely occur and should be seen in consultation. Isolated tendon lacerations, with the exception of those sustained by the flexor hallucis longus, can be repaired by the primary care physician.

Ankle. Like the dorsum of the foot, the ankle is frequently injured in the industrial setting. The etiology is a slip or trip in 50% of situations. Most commonly, a blow from a moving object can cause soft tissue damage, and because of the exposed nature of the ankle above the shoe line, lacerations and burns are quite common. Fractures occur uncommonly 2–4% of the time. Aviator's astragalus is a fracture of the neck of the talus following a head-on crash, as originally described in British aircraft during World War I. Flexion from pressure of a rudder bar beneath the forefoot forces the talus against the anterior margin of the tibia. Early rehabilitation is essential, though it is important to note that there is often an extended period of pain following an ankle injury.

Protection and Prevention

Of foremost concern in the management of industrial foot injuries are protection and prevention. A steel toe cap capable of sustaining a force of 75 foot-pounds is the required style because 30–35% of industrial foot injuries are caused by falling objects (e.g., equipment or construction material). Currently, steel shanks are not mandatory in the United States. A number of puncture-proof materials are being constructed, but so far, no satisfactory device has been found. Other characteristics of sole design that are recommended include materials that are resistant to slippage and are nonconductive. Due to continuous use and exposure to destructive environmental conditions, a safety shoe's average life expectancy is about 6 months; it must then be replaced to be effective. In North America, safety shoes do not include a metatarsal shield, but steel and foundry workers and loggers and workers in the pulp and paper industry should have such shields. High boots do not decrease the frequency of lateral ankle injuries due to indirect trauma. The incidence of direct blunt trauma is, however, reduced.

In addition to use of proper footwear, a number of safety measures should be undertaken. The floor and the workplace should be kept as clean and dry as possible. Rubber matting, abrasive strips, and carpeting drastically reduce slippage. Removal of nail-ridden lumber markedly reduces puncture wounds. Specific problems inherent in each department must be addressed. For instance, proper precautions must be taken in handling of hot fluids or high-voltage lines. The amount of time that workers spend on their feet should be addressed, because prolonged standing or walking, even with a comfortable and well-fitted shoe, can produce fatigue, backache, and calluses and can also lead to an accident. Consideration for safety must extend to the home environment, where, more often than not, the use of safety equipment stops because the individual leaves the work environment. A major offender at home is the power lawn mower. Regular use of steel-toe safety shoes can prevent the majority of such injuries. Less commonly, but equally dangerous, is the chain saw. Poor visualization, inadequate footwear,

and improper technique are the usual villains in such accidents.

SPORTS INJURIES

The physical forces and stress on the tissues of the foot and ankle are increased two to three times during athletic activities. However, most foot and ankle injuries are not unique to sports: they are just more common. The ankle sprain is probably the single most common sports injury. Aside from structural or biomechanical abnormalities, the most common etiologies of sports-related injuries to the foot and ankle are (1) rapid or improper warm-up, (2) overuse or excessive training, (3) overly intense workouts, (4) improper footwear, and (5) hard playing surfaces. In addition to the routine history and physical examination, sports-related questions should be asked to elicit the above information: What sports do you play? What is your warm-up or stretch routine? How often do you play? How long do you play? What type of athletic shoes do you wear? What surfaces do you play on? Once the etiology is determined, the patient may have to be instructed to modify the training routine or change sports in order to avoid further injury. The goal of treatment is to get the athlete back to the playing field as rapidly as possible and to avoid reinjury.

Black Toe or Runner's Toe

This condition is caused by increased pressure or friction to the toenail, leading to a subungual hematoma, partial nail avulsion, or both. Symptoms include pain and burning. Clinical signs are a black or purple toenail, with or without lifting of the distal aspect of the toenail. Treatment consists of drainage of the subungual hematoma (see Chapter 5), NSAIDs, and soaks as needed. Also, the patient should be instructed to check his or her athletic shoes for proper size and adequate toe box to avoid further injuries.

Black Heel

This condition, also termed calcaneal petechiae pseudochromadrosis plantaris, or jumper's or tennis heel, is characterized by variable coalescence of punctate, black dots, which appear suddenly on the sides of the heels. It usually affects people who jump (e.g., tennis and backetball players). The discoloration is not blood but rather contains melanin and a protein and is located at the orifice of the eccrine glands. Treatment is conservative and consists of adequate felt padding or a similar orthotic. The differential diagnosis should include examination not only for bleeding and coagulation but also for other sources of localized trauma and infection.

Blisters

Blisters are commonly caused by a repetitive sheer force. Symptoms include pain and tenderness. Clinical signs are weeping and bullae filled with clear fluid. Treatment consists of draining the bullae by needle puncture or aspiration, and leaving the roof of the bullae intact. However, if the blister has already ruptured, the roof should be debrided and the area covered with thin aseptic dressing. The athlete should be instructed to wear either two pairs of athletic socks or a pair of double-layered socks (Runique) to decrease the amount of friction in future activities or to apply moleskin ("second skin") tape, skin lubricant, or skin-hardening solutions (10% tannic acid or 3% saltwater).

Sprains of the Ankle

Sprains are ligamentous tears caused by forced overstretching or direct trauma. There are generally three classes of sprains based on severity: grade I (mild—less than 20% of fibers torn), grade II (moderate—20-70% of fibers torn), and grade III (severe—more than 70% of fibers torn) (Table 3). Although the grades are based on clinical findings and the results of diagnostic tests and radiographs, the grading is, nonetheless, somewhat of a subjective exercise.

Eighty-five percent of all ankle sprains occur to the lateral collateral ligaments during plantar inversion. The usual scenario consists of an athlete who has been running (e.g., during football or basketball) or skiing and who changes course in the direction of the ankle in question, either losing balance or being disturbed by an external force that results in marked supination (Fig. 11). In 85% of situations, the anterior talofibular ligament is injured, which represents 65% of all ankle sprains. With continued force in external leg rotation, supination, and mild dorsiflexion, the calcaneal fibular ligament will also be injured.

TABLE 3. *Diagnosis and Management of Ankle Sprains*

	Grade I	Grade II	Grade III
Lateral ligament	Anterior talofibular	Anterior talofibular, calcaneal fibular	Anterior talofibular, calcaneal fibular, posttalofibular
Medial ligament	Deltoid ligament—superficial	Deltoid ligament—superficial	Deltoid ligament—deep
Symptoms	Minimal pain and disability	Moderate pain and disability	Severe pain, significant functional loss
Weight bearing	Unimpaired	Difficult	Not possible
Signs	Slight edema, anterior drawer and talar tilt negative	Moderate edema, ecchymosis, anterior drawer and talar tilt positive	Severe edema, ecchymosis, anterior drawer and talar tilt positive, x-rays may show avulsion fracture
Stress films	Negative	Talar tilt 5-10 degrees, anterior drawer 4-14 mm	Talar tilt >20 degrees, anterior drawer >15 mm
Initial treatment	RICE, non-weight-bearing, posterior splint or air cast, NSAIDs, and analgesics as needed		
Long-term care	Weight-bearing brace or strapping for 2-3 wks, physical therapy for 1-2 wks	Unna boot, Jones compression bandage, weight bearing with post-operative shoe 2-4 wks orthotics/strapping 1-2 wks, physical therapy 2-4 wks	Weight-bearting short leg cast for 3-6 wks, then orthotics/strapping for 2-4 wks, physical therapy 4-6 wks, surgery

NSAIDs = nonsteroidal anti-inflammatory drugs; RICE = rest, ice and immobilization, compression, and elevation.

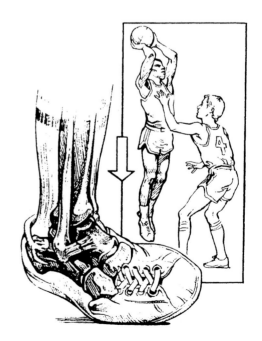

FIGURE 11. Spraining of the anterior talofibular ligament following forced plantarflexion and inversion.

Twenty percent of all ankle sprains represent combined injury to these ligaments. The posterior talofibular ligament is injured in 1% of cases due to further forced dorsiflexion.

Clinical Presentation. A careful history will probably elicit description of a twisting motion applied to the weight-bearing joint usually in association with internal rotation, adduction, and flipping of the foot under the ankle. Such relatively low-force activities such as running, walking, or stepping off a curb is typically recalled; the mechanism of injury in high-velocity competitive conditions is often unknown. The athlete usually complains of a sudden, intense, localized transient pain. Three quarters of patients will be able to bear weight on the injured ankle, and one third will discuss a history of previous sprains.

Unless it is seen during the golden period, the degree of edema generally increases with time and may involve the entire ankle. Grade II and III sprains are characterized by hemarthrosis in 60–70% of cases, and ecchymosis in 50–60% 24 hours after injury. The edema and distortion tend to be more severe in individuals who continue to be physically active following their injury. Although the area of ligamentous injury is always tender, 30–45% of patients complain of tenderness in uninjured adjoining ligaments. Thus, palpation should always begin in the injured ankle at a point farthest from the suspected site of injury. The examiner should remember always to compare the clinical findings with the normal side. In addition to evaluating individual ligaments by palpation, the clinician should check the integrity of the fibula and tibia. Point tenderness or crepitus should raise the suspicion of an associated fracture. Active range of motion, particularly that which reproduces the mechanism of injury, will predictably reproduce pain. This can be confirmed by passive range of motion and stress testing.

Inversion/Internal Rotation Injuries. Evidence of instability with lateral stress and plantar flexion not in the neutral position (i.e., an abnormal talar tilt) indicates a tear of the anterior talofibular ligament only. Tears of both the anterior talofibular ligament and the calcaneal fibular ligament are suggested by instability, with lateral stress in both plantar flexion and neutral positions. The anterior drawer test will demonstrate anterior displacement in tears of the anterior talofibular ligament. If there is clinical suspicion of an anterior talofibular ligament, but the drawer test is negative, inversion stress films should

be taken in both the neutral and plantarflexed positions. Increased amounts of talar tilt in plantar flexion with no increase in the neutral position indicate an isolated tear of the anterior talofibular ligament. Increased talar tilt of greater than 5–10 degrees in both the plantarflexion and neutral positions when compared with the normal side is suggestive of the tearing of both the anterior talofibular and the calcaneal fibular ligaments.

A consultation is advised for recurrent sprains and grade III injuries. The athlete may begin training again when strength and function of the injured side are equal to those of the uninjured side. An elastic ankle support, basket-weave strapping, or orthotic should be used for the first 2 weeks of training. In cases in which pain is present for months after the injury, a talar dome fracture must be ruled out by CT scan.

Medial Ankle Sprains. Ten to 15% of ankle sprains involve the medial collateral or tibiofibular ligament complexes. A sharp cut away from the involved ankle with severe pronation of the foot and internal leg rotation constitutes the usual mechanism of injury. Initially, the anterior portion of the superficial deltoid ligament (i.e., the tibial navicular ligament), the anteriomedial capsule, and the anterior smaller portion of the deep deltoid are involved. The mortise remains stable. With progressively more stress, sequential injuries occur to the anterior inferior tibiofibular ligament, the interosseous membrane and ligament, the remaining portions of the superficial deltoid ligament, and the deep deltoid ligament (i.e., the inferior transverse ligament and the posterior inferior tibiofibular ligament), resulting in complete separation of the tibia and fibula. A medial sprain in generally more severe than a lateral injury.

Medial stress films are used to assess the integrity of the deltoid ligament complex. Widening of the space between the talus and medial malleolus of greather than 2 mm indicates an unstable tear of the deep deltoid ligament. Separation of the distal tibia and fibula indicates a tear of the anterior-inferior tibiofibular ligament and interosseous ligament. Similarly, an anterior displacement of greater than 3 mm indicates a complete tear of the anterior talofibular ligament during draw stress radiographs.

Treatment. A grade I sprain is indicated by the absence of functional or anatomic instability. Treatment is purely supportive and is aimed at rapid restoration of normal ankle motion and strength. The RICE regimen should be followed for the first 24-48 hours and thereafter as needed during the rehabilitation process. Crutches or a cane should be used if there is any swelling or pain on weight bearing. The cane should be used on the contralateral uninjured side; single crutches are not recommended. Active range-of-motion (ROM) exercises within the limits of pain should be encouraged once edema has subsided. This should be supplemented by passive ROM exercises and progressive resistive exercises (PREs). With an elastic bandage or neoprene inner tube in place, isometric strengthening exercises can also be used. Although complete anatomic healing requires 4-6 weeks, strength and ROM exercises usually permit return to play in 1-2 weeks. It is advisable to use adhesive surgical strapping in the competitive situation to strengthen the ankle.

The RICE regimen, which is usually continued for longer periods of time (48-72 hours), is also adequate for grade II sprains. To ensure immobilization, a posterior splint, and Unna boot, or adhesive surgical strapping may be applied with the ankle in approximately a 90-degree position until the edema and pain have subsided. Thereafter, weight bearing, ROM exercises, and PREs, together with supplemental adhesive strapping, are initiated and supplemented by ice water or contrast soaks in order to promote the rehabilitation process. Supplemental adhesive strapping should be utilized during training. Several weeks to months should be allowed for complete healing, and return to play should be initiated only after full ROM and strength have been restored. It should be noted that some practitioners prefer cast immobilization for short periods of time. Such an approach may be useful in unstable injuries, although its routine use in stable sprains results in a considerable amount of athletic deconditioning and disuse atrophy.

The ideal treatment for third-degree sprains (i.e., nonoperative vs. operative) remains a source of controversy. The grade II regimen or the application of a cast for 6 weeks followed by an additional 6 weeks of ankle protection (e.g., cane, crutches, or adhesive strapping) represents the nonoperative approach. The rehabilitation process (e.g., ROM exercise and PRE) begins after cast removal and is continued until full strength and ROM are achieved, which may require 3-6 months from the time of injury. Whereas conservative intervention is a recurrent problem for grade III

sprains of the lateral ligaments, significant tears of the deep deltoid require surgical intervention.

The operative approach for grade III ankle sprains consists of accurate anatomic reapposition of the torn ligaments and, in the case of the deep deltoid, is considered the best way to maximize joint function and restore ligament strength. Primary surgical intervention should occur within the first 7-10 postinjury days. A risk of postoperative complications exists, and secondary reconstructive repairs are always possible for patients who have significant chronic symptoms. Following surgery, management is similar to that of the nonoperative approach for about 3 months. Although the incidence of chronic ankle instability in patients treated by surgery is difficult to determine, it appears to be approximately 5%.

Several words of caution are necessary concerning the management of sprains. In general, it is best to err on the conservative side when it comes to diagnosis and to be liberal when it comes to treatment and rehabilitation. One of the greatest mistakes is to allow an athlete with a grade II sprain to return too early to competition and suffer reinjury or a grade III sprain. In addition to misdiagnosis, rehabilitation is most commonly overlooked as a priority area. Specific ankle exercises (eversion, inversion, flexion, and dorsiflexion) should be known and taught by the practitioner. Proper warm-up and the recommendation to use a high-topped shoe or sneaker for routine activity as well as for training should be a regular part of the physician's armamentarium. Serial evaluations are a good idea if the degree of injury is unclear. Finally, it is important to consider the patient's chronologic age and functional capacity when deciding the most appropriate therapy. Nonoperative approaches are usually appropriate for middle-aged individuals or occasional athletes, whereas surgery is reserved for the young active person or older competitive athlete.

Turf Toe and Toe Sprain

These are caused when the toe, usually the hallux, jams in the sneaker and hyperextends. Progression of the injury can result in a tear to the joint capsule. Symptoms include pain and decreased ROM at the metatarsophalangeal joint. Clinical signs include edema, ecchymosis, and tenderness at the metatarsophalangeal joint. RICE, taping, and strapping the toe in a plantarflexed position to avoid further hyperextension are recommended, along with a rigid-sole shoe to avoid dorsiflexion of the toe.

Hallux Limitus

This can result from the repetitive athletic trauma of jumping and running (see Chapter 6).

Tendon Injuries

Tendon injuries can involve the tendon itself and its sheath or peritenon. Trauma to the tendon produces strains, whereas inflammation of the peritenon leads to tendinitis, peritendinitis, or tenosynovitis.

Tendinitis. Extensor tendinitis is an inflammation of the dorsal tendons of the foot and is commonly caused by overuse, short warm-ups, or long workouts. The symptoms include pain on ROM (i.e., dorsiflexion/plantarflexion), decreased ROM, and/or crepitation on range of motion. The clinical signs consist of mild edema, tenderness on direct palpation, and pain upon muscle and tendon function testing. RICE, NSAIDs, and immobilization (e.g., strapping, Unna boot, Jones compression bandage) are the recommended treatments. Modification in training, in athletic shoe gear, or in both is advisable.

Achilles Tendinitis. Repeated microtrauma to the Achilles, caused by rigid-soled shoes, skater's or hiker's boots, faulty technique, or hard landings can cause inflammation of the tendon and its sheath due to prolonged slow friction over the tendon. Acutely, there is localized pain, pain on stair climbing, crepitus, direct tenderness, and erythema; chronically there can be marked fibrosis and calcification. The differential diagnosis should include bursitis, strain, and arthritis. Treatment for Achilles tendinitis is conservative, consisting of aspirin and NSAIDs in association with adequate periods of rest, heat application, adhesive strapping, and physical therapy for 1–3 weeks. Steroid injections are contraindicated, and consultation should be sought for truly refractive cases. Shoe modifications include cutting out the heel counter or wearing an open-back shoe. In less severe cases, a soft, cushioned heel lift accompanied by a decreased activity level suffices. In recalcitrant or severe cases, immobilization and nonweightbearing are in order.

Posterior Tibial Tendinitis. This condition is caused by repetitive microtrauma during the pronation phase of running, cutting, jumping, and so on. Symptoms include pain inferior to the medial malleolus and decreased ROM. Clinical signs consist of edema and tenderness behind the medial malleolus or proximal to its insertion on the navicular tubercle; the pain is increased by inversion against resistance. Treatment varies according to the degree of the symptoms. Initially, RICE, NSAIDs, and analgesics are recommended as needed. For the long term, nonweightbearing and a short leg cast with the foot in inversion for 2–4 weeks, followed by medial posted orthosis, can also be helpful.

Peroneal Subluxation/Dislocation. The peroneal retinaculum can be torn by a direct blow to the back of the lateral malleolus while the tendons are taut in eversion and dorsiflexion. Powerful contraction of the peroneal muscles, particularly in maximal dorsiflexion, occurs most often in wrestling and downhill or cross-country skiing. Acute subluxation of the peroneal tendon is relatively uncommon and is most often confused with simple lateral ligament sprains. The tenderness and swelling, however, are centered behind the lateral malleolus and extend proximally over the tendons. They are absent over the anterolateral ankle capsule, where they would usually be found in a typical lateral sprain. One or both of the peroneal tendons may pop out of the groove onto the lateral aspect of the malleolus. Reduction is usually spontaneous. Differential diagnosis should include an ankle sprain, a contusion, and tenosynovitis. Palpation reveals direct tenderness over the tendons, which may be confused with tenosynovitis. With acute dislocation it is not possible to displace the tendon during examination. Treatment consists in relocation, if necessary by directing pressure on the tendon posteriorly and then casting the ankle in slight pronation and flexion. The plaster should be carefully and firmly molded to the contour of the lateral malleolus or a J-shaped piece of felt used to compress the tendon in place. Surgery should be considered for failed conservative therapy or for the serious athlete for whom lost time would be critical.

Untreated acute episodes or congenital weakness will result in chronic or recurrent subluxation of the peroneal tendons. There is usually a history of acute injury with appreciable soreness for many weeks followed by the recurrent feeling of something slipping out of place at the posterior portion of the ankle during foot eversion. There may be sharp pain and considerable stress noted with the condition. On physical examination, the retinaculum is usually thickened and the groove shallow. It is often possible to sublux or dislocate the tendons manually. Once again, treatment is surgical.

Rupture of the Achilles Tendon. This rupture can be caused by sudden dorsiflexion of a plantarflexed foot, sudden dorsiflexion of the ankle, pushing off the weight-bearing foot with the knee locked and extended, or a direct blow. Symptoms include sudden calf pain associated with audible snap, followed by antalgia and difficulty tiptoeing and climbing. The pain may be inconsistent with the degree of injury. Clinical signs consist of a positive Thompson-Doherty squeeze test (see p. 20), positive heel resistance test (easy dorsiflexion of the heel and foot against plantarflexion), and positive gap sign (palpable gap in tendon, which may be absent if edema is significant). Treatment varies with severity of injury, length of time between diagnosis and treatment, and age of the patient. Nonoperative treatment consists of RICE, NSAIDs and analgesics, nonweightbearing, a long leg gravity equinus cast for 6 weeks followed by a short-leg equinus cast for 2 weeks, and then a short walking cast for 2 weeks. Operative treatment should be considered in the serious athlete, and a specialist should be consulted.

Strains of the Ankle

Because the ankle is subject to large static and dynamic forces, strains of the joint are very common in a wide variety of sports. Strains may be classified in a similar fashion as sprains. The ankle joint per se is not involved in strains. The simple switching from street shoes that have a firm medial support and heel with a strong contour to an athletic shoe that has no heel, minimal support, and weak contour can cause a static strain of the tibial muscle. Medial strains involve the tibialis anterior, whereas the tibialis posterior is usually vulnerable at its attachment to the tuberosity of the naviculus or under its medial side due to its dual roles in effecting inversion and plantarflexion and supporting the foot arch. Tenderness will usually be palpable at the medial border of the arch with some spread under the arch and the back of the medial malleolus. The Achilles tendon can be strained at its site of attachment to the calcaneus, along the tendon's course, or most frequently at the musculotendinous junction. It is usually associated with tenosynovitis. Stronger forces in a middle-aged weekend athlete, particularly a forceful drive, push-off, or landing in forceful dorsiflexion such as in basketball, racquet sports, or broad jumping can result in spontaneous rupture of the tendon. The differential diagnosis should include strain of the calf musculature, contusion, or ankle sprain. The individual may often complain of a sensation of being accidentally kicked or struck by a ball in the back of the calf. A slight limp may be noted on examination, with variable amounts of edema and tenderness on palpation. During the golden period, a palpable gap will be noted, and the Thompson squeeze test will be positive. If the injury is seen several hours after the trauma occurred, swelling may obscure the gap. Active ROM will still preserve plantarflexion due to intact peroneal, tibial, and toe flexor muscle groups. For younger active individuals, surgical repair is indicated. Nonoperative results are usually excellent and are reserved for the older athlete whose primary interests are return to work and everyday routine activities rather than athletic performance.

Sesamoiditis is commonly caused by overuse of the foot in a plantarflexed position (e.g., sprinting). Symptoms include pain upon ambulation in and out of shoes and sub-first metatarsal pain. Clinical signs consist of pain upon dorsiflexion of the hallux, pain upon direct palpation of the sesamoid, and mild edema. X-ray evaluation to rule out fracture of the sesamoid is advised. RICE, NSAIDs, orthotic devices, and physical therapy are conservative methods of treatment. Surgical excision is rarely required.

Tibiotalar Impingement Syndrome

Repetitive microtrauma can lead to anterior or posterior impingement syndrome. The anterior aspect of the tibia hits against the talus during deep knee bends or "drive-off" from the planted foot (forced dorsiflexion) such as in football, rugby, or dancing. The posterior aspect of the tibia hits the posterior lateral tubercle of the talus during full weight bearing in maximum plantarflexion. Symptoms include vague anterolateral or posterolateral pain with extreme dorsiflexion during running or with plantarflexion during jumping, respectively.

The clinical signs for anterior impingement syndrome include point tenderness and edema over the anterior ankle and decreased dorsiflexion that produces pain. In posterior impingement, there is posterolateral tenderness, particularly with forced passive plantarflexion. Radiographs will visualize the spur and subchondral sclerosis and pseudocysts if there are degenerative changes. Treatment is the same for both syndromes; initially, RICE, NSAIDs, and analgesics are used as needed. Long-term treatment includes modification of activities, appropriate stretching, injection of long-acting and short-acting corticosteroids with lidocaine, and surgical excision for refractory cases.

BIBLIOGRAPHY

1. Birrer RB: Ankle injuries and the family physician. J Am Board Fam Pract 1:274–281, 1988.
2. Brackenbury PH, Muwanga C: A comparative double blind study of amoxicillin/clavulanate vs. placebo in the prevention of infection after animal bites. Arch Emerg Med 6:251, 1989.
3. Chisholm CD, Schlesser JF: Plantar puncture wounds: Controversies and treatment recommendations. Am Emerg Med 18:1352–1357, 1989.
4. Cracehiolo A III: Office treatment of adult foot problems. Orthop Clin North Am 13:511–524, 1982.
5. Crawford AH, Gabriel KR: Foot and ankle problems. Orthop Clin North Am 18:649–666, 1987.
6. Davis AW, Alexander IJ: Problematic fractures and dislocations in the foot and ankle of athletes. Clin Sports Med 9:163–181, 1990.
7. Forrester DM, Kerr R: Trauma to the foot. Radiol Clin North Am 28:423–433, 1990.
8. Frey CC, Shereff MJ: Tendon injuries about the ankle in athletes. Clin Sports Med 7:103–118, 1988.
9. Garfinkel D, Rothenberger LA: Foot problems in athletes. J Fam Pract 19:239–250, 1984.
10. Garrick JG, Requa RK: The epidemiology of foot and ankle injuries in sports. Clin Sports Med 7:29–36, 1988.
11. Hawkins BJ, Haddad RJ Jr: Hallux rigidus. Clin Sports Med 7:37–49, 1988.
12. Lassiter TE, Malone TR, Garrett WE: Injury to the lateral ligaments of the ankle. Orthop Clin North Am 20:629–640, 1989.
13. McBryde AM, Anderson RB: Sesamoid foot problems in the athlete. Clin Sports Med 7:51–60, 1988.
14. Paley D, Hall H: Calcaneal fracture controversies: Can we put Humpty Dumpty together again? Orthop Clin North Am 20:665–678, 1989.
15. Perlman MD, Leveille D, Gale B: Traumatic classification of the foot and ankle. J Foot Surg 28:551–585, 1989.
16. Resnick CD, et al: Puncture wounds: Therapeutic considerations and a new classification. J Foot Surg 29:147–153, 1990.
17. Wojtys EM: Sports injuries in the immature athlete. Orthop Clin North Am 18:689–708, 1987.

Chapter 14

GOUT

Richard B. Birrer, M.D.

Gout is characterized by an elevated serum level of uric acid, the deposition of monosodium urate crystals in and around a number of tissues, and subsequent recurrence of attacks of acute arthritis, renal disease, and urolithiasis. Originally derived from the Latin word gutta, meaning "drop," gout was described centuries before the common era. Hippocrates used the word podagra, which comes from the Greek meaning "foot attack." Traditionally, gout has affected the affluent and prestigious, notably Alexander the Great, Benjamin Franklin, William Harvey, Isaac Newton, and Cardinal Wolsey. At least 50% of patients have a positive family history of the disease, and, though it is more common in men, women who carry the trait usually develop the disease several years after menopause.

Classically, a gouty attack begins during the early hours of the morning, usually affecting a single joint, particularly the first metatarsophalangeal joint in 75% of cases.

PATHOGENESIS

The biomechanical hallmark of gout is hyperuricemia, which is present at some point in up to 98% of patients with the disease. The uric acid level may not be elevated in all patients during an acute attack, however. Gout may be a primary metabolic disease due to an inborn error in the intermediary metabolism of purines and related compounds, or it may be secondary due to the excessive degradation of the nucleoproteins in nucleic acids, as occurs in some hematologic disorders or drug side effects. In individuals with primary gout, the total miscible uric acid pool is greatly

enlarged, particularly among those with tophaceous gout. As a result, the majority of dietary nitrogen is excreted as uric acid and not as urea. The increased uric acid pool is due either to the decreased renal clearance of urate, presumably due to the defect in tubular reabsorption and/or tubular secretion, or to increased production of urate through the biosynthesis of purines or the excessive ingestion of dietary purines. Causes of secondary gout include polycythemia rubra vera, the leukemias, and any large tumor mass that is lysed by chemotherapy or radiotherapy. Drugs such as diuretics and low-dose aspirin also may induce hyperuricemia, most likely by blocking the tubular reabsorption of uric acid. Predisposing factors to a gouty attack include dietary and alcohol indiscretions and the ingestion of organ meats. Sometimes a small injury may provoke a gouty attack.

PATHOLOGY

Urate crystals are deposited in the synovial membrane, articular cartilage, joint capsule, subarticular and juxta-articular bone, and surrounding soft tissue (Fig. 1). The inflammatory process begins with the ingestion of urate crystals by polymorphonuclear leukocytes that have been attracted by the activation of the complement cascade and kinin system. The leukocytes are degranulated due to their inability to degrade the crystals. The result is lysis of the white cell membrane, death of the cell, and release of lysosomal enzymes that initiate the inflammatory reactions characteristic of the topical gouty attack. Intense pain, swelling, erythema, and warmth occur due to

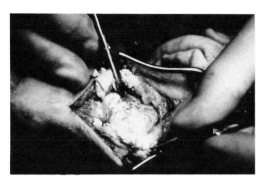

FIGURE 1. Gouty crystals deposited in first metatarsophalangeal joint.

surrounding cell necrosis. The entire articular surface and subchondral bone can be destroyed and urate crystals deposited in soft connective tissue forming tophi, particularly in the bursae, ligaments, tendons, and subcutaneous layers of the skin. Though the first metatarsophalangeal joint is the most common area for the presentation of a gouty attack, the ankle, fingers, heel, lesser toes, and knee may also become involved.

CLINICAL MANIFESTATIONS

An attack of gouty arthritis is intermittent and asymmetric. Usually the attack appears suddenly and resolves spontaneously over 72-96 hours. The ensuing asymptomatic period may last from several days to years. The pain of an acute attack progressively increases in intensity in the first 24 hours, followed by edema, warmth, and erythema. The pain tends to be gnawing and throbbing in nature and may be so severe as to prevent walking and necessitate the removal of all clothing and footwear from the affected area. There may be systemic fever during the attack. Seventy-five to 80% of cases involve a monoarticular arthritis of the metatarsophalangeal joint in the first toe (Fig. 2). Ten to 20% of patients may have an oligoarthritis or polyarthritis even during the first attack.

Though the diagnosis of gout is frequently made both clinically and by the finding of an elevated serum level of uric acid, demonstration of the characteristic monosodium monohydrate crystals in the synovial fluid is pathognomonic. A tuberculin or insulin syringe with a 22-23 gauge needle can be used to enter the joint aseptically and aspirate a small amount of synovial fluid. (Preloading the syringe with a small amount of sterile saline is not recommended, because water-containing solutions often dissolve the urate crystals.) The aspirate should then be observed under an ordinary light microscope to determine whether there are crystals present. If crystals are present, the examination should be performed with a compensated polarizing light microscope to determine the crystal type. Urate crystals are characteristically needle shaped and produce strong negative birefringence. The crystals of pseudogout (e.g., calcium pyrophosphate arthropathy, chondrocalcinosis, pseudopodagra) demonstrate weak positive birefringence and, unlike urate crystals, are radiopaque and rhomboid in shape.

Pseudogout can involve the first metatarsophalangeal joint and should be considered part of the differential diagnosis of any inflamed joint. Chronic tophaceous gout can also affect the foot and usually appears after an undetermined period of gout that has been either not treated or treated ineffectively.

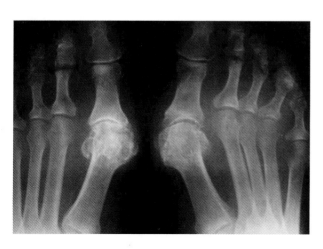

FIGURE 2. X-ray shows arthritic changes at first metatarsophalangeal joint secondary to gout.

Tophaceous gout tends to present as a symmetric polyarthritis and may involve any area of the body but most frequently the extensor surface of the hand and elbow, the first metatarsophalangeal joint, the heel (particularly the Achilles tendon), and the ear. Clinical suspicion must be confirmed by aspiration of the nodule and examination of the material for crystals.

TREATMENT

The therapeutic management of gout is twofold: treatment of the acute attack and long-term prevention of both further acute attacks and the development of chronic tophaceous gout. Several medications can be used for the acute attack. Most commonly, colchicine is recommended. It appears to act by inhibiting microtubule function of the polymorphonuclear leukocytes, thus reducing their mobility and phagocytic activity. The usual dosage of colchicine consists of two tablets initially (1–1.2 mg) followed by one tablet every 2 hours or until there is relief of joint pain or the patient develops severe nausea, vomiting, or diarrhea. Clinical response to colchicine is usually seen in 8–12 hours, although gout is the only disorder that consistently responds to the drug and, therefore, is considered a diagnostic test. In order to avoid gastrointestinal side effects as well as to produce a clinical response in 6–8 hours, colchicine can be administered intravenously slowly in a dosage of 2–3 mg. It is imperative that the medication be given with the utmost care, as extravasation can cause local tissue necrosis. One to two tablets of the drug can be prophylactically administered following the acute attack. Other medications include NSAIDs (e.g., ibuprofen, 600 mg three or four times daily for several days, indomethacin, 25–50 mg three or four times daily for several days, or phenylbutazone, 200 mg every 4 hours for 2–3 days). An acute attack of pseudogout is best treated with an NSAID.

The treatment of tophaceous gout and chronic gouty arthritis often consists of a combined pharmacological and surgical approach. Elevated levels of serum uric acid can be reduced by increasing uric acid excretion through inhibition of renal tubular resorption by using uricosuric agents such as probenecid 0.5 gm twice daily or sulfinpyrazone 100 mg twice daily. These agents are especially useful in preventing and ameliorating attacks of chronic gouty arthritis, preventing the formation of tophaceous deposits, and decreasing the size of tophi already present. Their effectiveness depends on satisfactory renal function. When the glomerular filtration rate falls below 20–30 ml/min, the agents become ineffective. Allopurinol, a potent inhibitor of xanthine oxidase, decreases serum and urinary uric acid levels by inhibiting uric acid formation. It is particularly useful in the presence of poor kidney function and is administered in a dosage of 100 mg two or three times daily. When used alone, it can affect the rate of disappearance of already existing tophi, and when used in combination with uricosuric agents, it can further prevent the formation of, as well as reduce the size of, existing tophi. Allopurinol should be initiated before uricosuric drugs if there is a danger of stone formation as in the case of a massive urate burden from leukemia of polycythemia.

Occasionally surgical management is required to remove tophaceous deposits that have not responded to medical therapy. A number of authors have recommended surgery for gout of the foot in the following situations.

1. Large tophi that compress adjacent nerves, vessels, and tendons; tophi present in weight-bearing areas; and tophi that interfere with wearing shoes.

2. A tophus with a draining sinus.

3. Painful destruction or deformity of the toe joints.

With the exception of tophi involving the superficial soft tissues, such surgery is not within the purview of the practicing family physician. Therefore, the patient should see a consultant. Superficial tophi are usually encapsulated by fibrous tissue and can be shelled out by careful dissection and curettage. Prophylactic colchicine should be initiated before a planned operation, because surgery can precipitate a gouty attack.

BIBLIOGRAPHY

1. Becker MA: Clinical aspects of monosodium urate monohydrate crystal deposition disease. Rheum Dis Clin North Am 14:377–394, 1988.
2. Egan R, et al: Radiographic features of gout in the foot. J Foot Surg 26:434–439, 1987.
3. German DC, et al: Hyperuricemia and gout. Med Clin North Am 70:419–436, 1986.
4. Wallace SL, et al: Therapy in gout. Rheum Dis Clin North Am 14:441–457, 1988.

Chapter 15

ARTHRITIS

Michael P. DellaCorte, D.P.M.

Arthritic conditions affecting the foot can be monoarticular, polyarticular, or migratory. The pain that the patient experiences can be caused by the joint itself or by any of the surrounding structures of the joint, such as the joint capsule or ligament. The incidence of degenerative joint disease (DJD) is much higher in patients with biomechanical abnormalities. Long-standing continuous trauma is a significant factor in the development of secondary DJD. Studies based on x-ray findings have shown the DJD is a ubiquitous condition that increases in frequency with age.

Rheumatoid arthritis (RA) is more prevalent in females than males in a ratio of nearly 3:1. The diagnosis is based on history, physical examination, blood work, and x-rays of the hands and the feet. Studies have shown that more than 3% of the population examined had some evidence of RA.

OSTEOARTHRITIS

Osteoarthritis has been termed the wear-and-tear arthritis. The prevalence of osteoarthritis in the feet is about 20% in the population ranging in age from 18 to 79 years. Women are affected more than men. The disease affects the bone, cartilage, and joint capsule but not the synovial lining. It is, therefore, technically not an inflammatory arthritis, but the surrounding joint structures can become inflamed and painful. The condition progresses in a cycle.

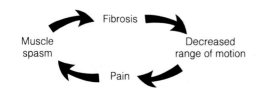

Pain in the joint or in the surrounding joint structures causes spasm and burning. The subsequent fibrosis and stiffening of the joint structures decrease range of motion (ROM) and cause more pain. A joint that is not biomechanically ideal in function or that has been traumatized leads to progressive degeneration of the articular cartilage.

The clinical manifestations of aching, burning, and spasm are usually relieved by rest. Symptoms may be out of proportion compared with the clinical evaluation. Physical findings consist of deformed joints with crepitus and pain noted on movement. There may be localized tenderness of the underlying joint capsule. ROM is generally decreased, and there may be some clinical deformities such as bunions, hammer toes, bone spurs, and so on. The diagnosis is made by consideration of the patient's age, the gradual onset of the symptoms, the clinical presentation of the joint, and radiographic findings (Fig. 1), that is, uneven joint narrowing, subchondral sclerosis, hypertrophic bone changes, and spur formation. Joint aspiration and fluid analysis are rarely necessary but reveal a noninflammatory picture (Table 1). The differential diagnosis includes gout, traumatic arthritis, and seronegative and seropositive disorders.

Treatment consists of nonsteroidal anti-inflammatory drugs (NSAIDs), injection therapy (two to four times per year), physiotherapy, and orthotic control of any abnormal foot function contributing to the arthritis. The padding of painful bone prominences with ¼-inch felt may also give temporary relief. Molded shoes to accommodate for bony prominences will help on a long-term basis. Athletic running shoes (i.e., sneakers) often help to relieve the pain of osteoarthritis and improve function. The goal of treatment is to break the pain cycle. Surgical intervention, consisting of arthroplasties, joint replacements, or both (Fig. 2) should be considered if symptoms do not resolve in 3–6 months. A specialist should be consulted.

RHEUMATOID ARTHRITIS

Rheumatoid arthritis (RA) is a systemic disease with inflammatory changes throughout the connective tissue of the body. The foot is the initial site of RA in

TABLE 1. *Nonsteroidal Anti-Inflammatory Drugs (NSAIDs)*

Class	Availability (mg)	Doses per Day	Maximum Dosage (mg)
Propionic acids			
Fenoprofen	200, 300, 600	3 or 4	3,200
Flubiprofen	50,100	2–4	300
Ibuprofen	200, 300, 400, 600, 800	3 or 4	3,200
Ketoprofen	25, 50, 75	3 or 4	300
Naproxen	250, 375, 500, 125/5 ml	2 or 3	1,500
Naproxen sodium	275, 500	3	1,375
Indoles			
Indomethacin	10, 25, 50, 75, 25/5 ml	2–4	200
Sulindac	150, 200	2	400
Tolmetin	200, 400	3 or 4	2,000
Fenamates			
Meclofenamate	50,100	4	400
Mefenamic acid	250	4	1,000
Oxicams			
Piroxicam	10, 20	1	20
Phenylacetic acids			
Diclofenac sodium	25, 50, 75	4	200
Salicylates			
Diflunisal	250, 500	2 or 3	1,500

If clinical response is not seen after 3–4 weeks of treatment, another drug from a different class should be considered.

WARNINGS
Hypersensitivity reactions
   Anaphalactoid reaction among patients allergic to aspirin
Gastrointestinal effects
   Serious gastrointestinal toxicity such as bleeding, ulceration, and perforation can occur at any time, with or without warnings or symptoms, in patients treated with NSAIDs long term. Contraindicated in patients with peptic ulcer.
Central nervous system effects
   Indomethacin may aggravate depression, other psychiatric disturbances, epilepsy, and parkinsonism, and therefore must be used with caution. Headaches are also quite common.
Renal effects
   Many forms of renal dysfunction occur due to prostaglandin inhibition. Contraindicated in renally impaired patients. May decrease the effects of diuretics and therefore must be used with caution in hypertensive and cardiac patients. Sulindac is least likely to cause acute renal dysfunction.
Miscellaneous
   Safety of drugs not established in pregnancy; they are excreted in breast milk. Must be used with caution among elderly patients more prone to adverse effects. Tolmetin and naproxen are the only drugs labeled for treatment of juvenile arthritis; safety of remainder of drugs for use in children has not been established; not recommended for children less than 14 years old.

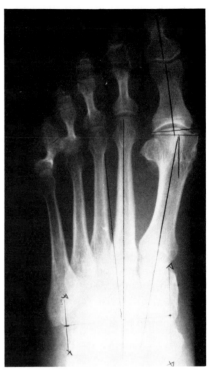

FIGURE 1. Osteoarthritis of first metatarsophalangeal joint with uneven joint narrowing, spur formation, and subchondral sclerosis.

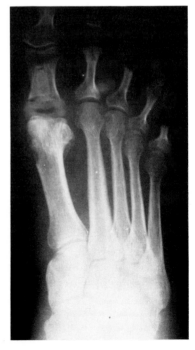

FIGURE 2. Total joint replacement for treatment of osteoarthritis.

12-20% of patients, but throughout the course of the disease, foot involvement may reach 90%. At the joint level, there is chronic proliferative inflammation of the synovial membrane that causes an irreversible change in the joint capsule and articular cartilage. These structures are replaced by granulation tissue. X-ray findings (Fig. 3) consist of uniform joint narrowing, bone atrophy, bone erosion, punched-out areas in the joint, and subluxed deformed joints with bone resorption as in osteoporosis. The proximal interphalangeal joint and the metatarsal phalangeal joint are the most common joints affected in the foot (70-80%). The deformities are generally in the small joints of the feet, with subluxation and fibular deviation. The midtarsal joint (65%) and the subtalar joint (35%) can also be affected in RA, leading to a flatfoot deformity. The diagnosis is made if one to five of the following criteria are present for at least 6 weeks.

1. Morning stiffness lasting more than ½ hour
2. Pain on motion or tenderness in at least one joint
3. Swelling of at least one joint
4. Swelling of at least one other joint
5. Symmetrical joint swelling with simultaneous involvement of the same joint on both sides of the body except proximal interphalangeal joints
6. Subcutaneous nodules
7. X-ray changes typical of RA
8. Positive latex fixation test (RA factor)
9. Precipitate from synovial fluid
10. Characteristic histologic changes in synovial membrane
11. Characteristic histologic changes in nodules showing granulomatous foci and so on

There are usually accompanying systemic findings of fever, weight loss, fatigue, and anorexia. An inflammatory picture is found on joint aspiration and fluid analysis (see Table 1). Definite rheumatoid arthritis is diagnosed if five of the above criteria are present, and probable RA if the following are present for 3 weeks.

1. Tenderness or pain on ROM
2. Morning stiffness
3. History of joint swelling
4. Subcutaneous nodules
5. Elevated sedimentation rate or C-reactive protein
6. Iritis

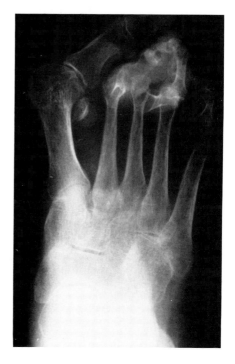

FIGURE 3. Rheumatoid arthritis—x-ray findings.

The lab tests for RA are as follows.

1. Complete blood count (there may be some changes in the white count with a shift to the left in acute cases)
2. Erythrocyte sedimentation rate (may be moderate to markedly increased)
3. RA test or latex fixation test (to determine if rheumatoid factor is present)
4. Uric acid (usually normal)
5. Synovial fluid analysis (to determine increased white blood cell count; may be cloudy with decreased viscosity)

TREATMENT

There is no specific or curative therapy for RA. Patients benefit from a combination of medical, surgical, and rehabilitative services. The goals in management are to suppress the joint and tissue inflammation, maintain function, an repair damaged joints surgically. Depending on the level of the disease, these goals can be accomplished by using medications such as NSAIDs. The more complex medical treatment regimens such as gold salts and steroids may warrant a rheumatology consultation. Intra-articular or periarticular infiltrations with corticosteroid and local anesthetic reduce inflammation at the local level. Debridement and padding of any hyperkeratotic lesions offer relief of underlying bursitis. Plastazote inserts, accommodative orthotics, and molded shoes give long-term relief. Running sneakers are also very helpful.

Once the arthritic changes have completely destroyed the cartilage and the joints of the forefoot have dislocated, surgical management should be considered (Fig. 4). Indications include painful calluses and corns, ulcerations at pressure points, severe pain when bearing weight, and painful hallux valgus. The classic procedure for an RA patient with a bunion and subluxed hammer toes at the metatarsophalangeal joint ranges from first metatarsophalangeal joint arthroplasty to arthrodesis and pan metatarsal head resection. This procedure is not cosmetic; it is purely accommodative. The recovery period may be prolonged, particularly if the patient is on steroid therapy. A cast and crutches for 4–6 weeks may constitute an inconvenience for these patients, especially if the arthritis has affected the hands. Rest and physiotherapy following surgery are mandatory. The prognosis is excellent for pain-free ambulation in normal shoe gear. Patients will have a shorter foot on the surgical side due to bone removal, and some modifications of shoe gear may be necessary.

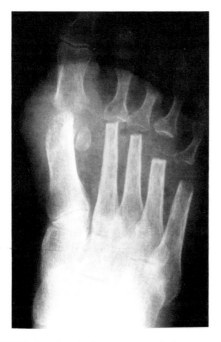

FIGURE 4. Surgical management of rheumatoid arthritic foot.

SERONEGATIVE DISORDERS

Seronegative disorders are arthritic conditions that do not have a positive rheumatoid factor in the blood. These include Reiter's syndrome and psoriatic arthritis.

Reiter's Syndrome

Reiter's syndrome is believed to be triggered by an infectious process in genetically susceptible individuals. The HLA B-27 surface antigen is both nondiagnostic and positive in these genetically predisposed individuals less than 50% of the time. The diagnosis is based on clinical evaluation and a triad of symptoms: conjunctivitis, urethritis, and arthritis. The arthritis affects primarily the lower extremity. It usually arises 1 week to 1 month after onset of the urethritis or enteric infection.

In the initial attack, the most commonly involved articulations, in order of decreasing frequency, are the knee or ankle, metatarsophalangeal joint, heel, shoulder, hip, and lumbar spine. There also may be digital involvement with synovitis and joint effusion that cause a swollen toe, sometimes called "sausage toe." The condition is generally self-limiting. Treatment is geared mainly toward patient comfort. NSAIDs and therapy consist of whirlpool baths, paraffin baths, and ultrasound work well to relieve symptoms.

Psoriatic Arthritis

Psoriatic arthritis affects up to 7% of patients with psoriasis. The patient must be diagnosed with psoriasis and have at least one psoriatic patch. The most common form of the arthritis is an asymmetric peripheral polyarthritis that affects primarily the distal interphalangeal joints. Other forms of this arthritis are very similar to RA. The psoriatic patient should have base line x-ray evaluation to evaluate the joints. Some of the x-ray findings are destructive arthritis at the distal interphalangeal joints of the hands and feet and bony ankylosis of the interphalangeal joints of the hands and feet. Resorption of the distal phalangeal tufts, the so-called "penciling" of the digit, is a classic sign of psoriatic arthritis. There is no specific treatment for psoriatic arthritis. Surgical intervention should be approached cautiously due to the Koebner phenomenon (i.e., the appearance of psoriatic lesions in areas of trauma or surgical incisions).

TABLE 2. *Examination of Joint Fluid*

	Clarity	Color	Viscosity	White Blood Cells (per cu mm)	Polymorpho-nuclear Leukocytes	Culture	Mucin Clot	Glucose	Differential Diagnosis
Normal	Transparent	Clear	High	<200	25%	Negative	Firm	Nearly equal to blood	—
Noninflammatory	Transparent	Yellow	High	200-2,000	25%	Negative	Firm	Nearly equal to blood	Degenerative joint disease Trauma[†] Osteochondritis dissecans Osteochondromatosis Neuropathic arthropathy Hypertrophic osteo-arthropathy Pigmented villonodular synovitis
Inflammatory	Translucent opaque	Yellow to opalescent	Low	2,000-100,000	50% or more	Negative	Friable	>25— lower than blood	Rheumatoid arthritis Gout and pseudogout Reiter's syndrome Ankylosing spondylitis Psoriatic arthritis Rheumatic fever Systemic lupus erythematosus Scleroderma
Septic	Opaque	Yellow to green	Variable	>100,000	75% or more[*]	Often positive	Friable	<25— much lower than blood	Bacterial infection

[*] Lower with infections caused by partially treated or low-virulence organisms.
[†] May be hemorrhagic.

SEPTIC ARTHRITIS

Joint infection may follow surgery or trauma. Joint sepsis accounts for 0.02% of hospital admissions and is a true medical emergency requiring early diagnosis and aggressive treatment. It is most commonly seen in children, the elderly, and patients with underlying systemic disease or a previously damaged joint. The clinical presentation is similar to gout and consists of a red, hot, swollen, painful joint. Cellulitis may or may not be present. Complete blood count, a chemistry panel, and radiographs of joints will help narrow the diagnosis. The definitive diagnosis of a septic joint is made by aspiration and analysis of the joint fluid (Table 2). The differential diagnosis includes other causes of inflammatory and noninflammatory arthritis. If an infection is suspected, the patient should be admitted to the hospital, blood cultures drawn, a broad-spectrum intravenous antibiotic administered (e.g., cephalosporin), and the joint incised and drained. Immediate diagnosis and treatment are essential for resumption of regular activity and joint function. The amount of joint damage is related to the severity and length of the infection.

BIBLIOGRAPHY

1. Coughlin MJ: The rheumatoid foot. Postgrad Med 75(5): 207-216, 1984.
2. Gilkes JJ: Skin and nail changes in the arthritic foot. Bailliere's Clin Rheumatol 1:335-354, 1987.
3. Hollander JL: Arthritis and Allied Conditions, 11th ed. Philadelphia, Lea & Febiger, 1988.
4. Kitaoka HB: Rheumatoid burdfoot. Orthop Clin North Am 20:593-604, 1989.
5. Rana NA: Juvenile rheumatoid arthritis of the foot. Foot Ankle 3:2, 1982.
6. Spector AK, Christman RA: Coexistent gout and rheumatoid arthritis. JAPMA 79:552-557, 1989.

Chapter 16

DIABETES

Daniel L. Picard, M.D., Caren B. Schumer, D.P.M.,
and Richard B. Birrer, M.D.

Five to 6% of the population of the United States suffers from diabetes mellitus. Because of the remarkable consequences of their disease, diabetics are vulnerable to foot complications. Rampant and often widespread arteriosclerosis of the lower extremities combined with peripheral neuropathy makes these patients susceptible to foot ulcerations, infection, and gangrene. Not uncommonly, a foot ulcer, a recurrent fungal infection, or a paronychial abscess will be the first clue to chemical or clinical diabetes.

The following facts illustrate the severity of diabetic complications in the lower extremities.

1. Gangrene of the lower extremities occurs 53 times as frequently in male diabetics and 71 times as frequently in female diabetics as in nondiabetics.

2. Fifty to 70% of all nontraumatic amputations are performed on diabetics.

3. Fifty percent of patients who had a unilateral amputation will develop a limb-threatening complication in the opposite extremity within 2 years of the amputation.

4. The 3-year survival rate for diabetics who have undergone amputation is only 50%.

5. Two billion dollars was spent in 1988 for hospital care related to diabetic amputations.

The need for an aggressive and multidisciplinary approach to prevent limb loss is of paramount importance and may reduce these figures by 50%.

PATHOPHYSIOLOGY

Angiopathy and neuropathy are the two pathologic processes that lead to the "diabetic foot."

Arterial Occlusive Disease

Diabetic patients display gross and microscopic pathology that is quite similar to nondiabetics with advanced arteriosclerosis. In the diabetic, it is, however, more widespread and more rapidly progressive. Diabetics are found to have microangiopathy that appears as intimal thickening, involving primarily the basement membrane. At an early stage, this thickening does not usually occlude the lumen but might impede the diffusion of nutrients through the capillary wall and limit the migration of leukocytes toward areas of infection. Diabetics appear to have more pronounced disease in the distal vasculature involving the metatarsal vessels three times as often as in nondiabetics.

Peripheral Neuropathy

Direct metabolic damage to the Schwann cell results in segmental loss of the myelin sheath. It is believed to be secondary to axonal degeneration that involves both small and large myelinated and unmyelinated fibers. Biochemical abnormalities include depletion of axonal inositol, accumulation of intraneural sorbitol, and impairment of intra-axonal vesicle transport. These changes predispose the diabetic patient to foot injury and infections.

Diabetic neuropathy encompasses a wide spectrum of neurologic conditions affecting sensory, motor, and autonomic functions. Symmetric polyneuropathy is classically described with a sock-glove distribution. Sensory impairment with loss of proprioception, loss of sense of touch and vibration, and loss of pain and temperature perception, usually precedes motor dysfunction. The latter affects the intrinsic muscles of the foot and leads to alteration in shape and a change in gait pattern. Lastly, autonomic nervous system abnormalities yield a picture analogous to sympathectomy: the foot is warm, dry, and susceptible to cracks and fissures. The biomechanical alterations that result from neuropathy, combined with a decrease in sensation, make the diabetic foot more prone to ulcerations and superinfection.

CLINICAL EVALUATION

The most important component in the evaluation of the diabetic foot is the clinical examination. A careful dermatologic, neurologic, orthopedic, and vascular examination must be performed to assess patients at risk for foot problems.

Dermatologic Examination

The lower extremity is by far the most commonly affected skin area in diabetes. Infections of the toenails, nail bed, and adjacent structures compose an important and frequently encountered group of problems in diabetic patients.

Onychomycosis is among the most common dermatologic manifestations in the diabetic foot. The fungal infection is recognized by its yellowish-white opaque appearance. It is, for the most part, asymptomatic; however, the nails become very thick; subungual ulceration can sometimes result from an increase in shoe pressure on the thickened nail. Often, the patient with mycotic nails has an associated chronic dermatophytosis (tinea pedis). The organisms that cause both the skin and nail infections are *Trichophyton mentagrophytes*, *Trichophyton rubrum*, and *Epidermophyton floccosum*. *Candida albicans* is less commonly found.

Onychocryptosis, or ingrowing nail, is a common and usually painful condition that may be aggravated by tight shoes and improper nail care. The inflamed nail fold must be addressed by excising the offending nail. Without immediate and proper attention, this can quickly develop into a paronychia, followed by cellulitis and sepsis.

The interstitial web spaces of the diabetic, particularly the fourth space, may become macerated and white. The differential diagnosis must include tinea pedis, moniliasis, white psoriasis, soft corns, and bacterial infections from single or mixed organisms such as Proteus, Corynebacterium, Bacillus, Staphylococcus, Bacteroides, Clostridium, and Pseudomonas. Cultures for fungi, candida, and aerobic and anaerobic bacteria are essential for diagnosis of nail and skin infections. Proper and immediate attention is necessary in order to prevent more serious sequelae.

Hyperkeratotic lesions are no more frequent in the diabetic than the nondiabetic. However, such lesions in the ischemic or neuropathic foot can, if left untreated, lead to subkeratotic ulcerations, hematomas, and sinus tracts. As the pressure increases, the microcirculation becomes impeded and frank ulceration occurs.

Many other cutaneous lesions associated with diabetes also present in the lower extremity. Granuloma annulare, idiopathic hemorrhagic bullae, xanthochromia, xanthoma, and necrobiosis lipoidica diabeticorum should raise the clinician's suspicion of underlying diabetes. Pruritus is a common finding due to dryness of skin that results from autonomic dysfunction.

Neurologic Examination

Neuropathy develops slowly, initially consisting of paresthesias and night cramps and progressing to a loss of vibration sense, loss of perception of pain and light touch, and, finally, loss of deep tendon reflexes. These clinical findings are a reflection of the fact that the more distal portion of the nerve exhibits greater demyelinization than the proximal portion. Evidence of peripheral autonomic dysfunction is exhibited by a brittle keratosis, atrophy of the fat pads, and loss of sebaceous gland function.

Because motor nerves are also involved, diabetics often develop a weakness in the intrinsic muscles of the feet, leading to a disruption of the normal fine balance between the toe flexors and extensors. The result is hammer toe deformities with extensor subluxation of toes with concomitant plantar prominence of the metatarsal heads and proximal migration of the metatarsal fat pads. Weight bearing shifts to the unprotected metatarsal heads, and the now more prominent dorsally contracted toes are impacted into the shoe. In response to the trauma, the body reacts by producing excessive amounts of hyperkeratotic tissue or corns (heloma dura) and calluses (tylomata).

In addition to these structural changes, severe long-standing neuropathy can lead to a neuropathic arthropathy or Charcot joint. Due to the loss of proprioceptive sense, excessive and abnormal ranges of motion can develop in a joint. The result is a tearing of supportive ligaments and soft tissue, destruction of the joint cartilage, and microfractures of bone. The foot may appear grossly deformed, with typical rocker-bottom subluxation of the midtarsal region or subluxation of the metatarsophalangeal joints. In an acute Charcot joint, the foot will be erythematous and quite warm to the touch and show signs of anhidrosis. Almost always the pulses are bounding and the patient supplies a history describing relatively mild to absent pain.

Orthopedic Examination

The importance of recognizing areas of potential breakdown due to altered weight-bearing patterns and bony prominences cannot be overemphasized. After observation of gait pattern, structural deformities must be assessed. Hallux valgus deformity can lead to ulceration of the medial eminence; hallux rigidus or degenerative joint disease of the first metatarsophalangeal joint can lead to excessive motion and ulceration at the distal interphalangeal joint of the hallux. Hammer-toe and claw-toe deformities can lead to ulcerations at the proximal interphalangeal joint, the distal interphalangeal joint, or both. Prominent metatarsal heads lead to hyperkeratotic tissue and thus predispose to plantar ulcerations. A rocker-bottom or Charcot foot, characteristically appearing as a dorsiflexed and abducted forefoot, tends to cause midfoot plantar ulcerations. Patients with prior amputations will also have altered weight bearing and areas of increased pressure predisposing to breakdown. Collectively, the neuropathic, angiopathic, and structural changes, together with the defects in the skin barrier, wound-healing chemotaxis, and phagocytosis, predispose the diabetic foot to easy and often serious infection.

Vascular Examination

Assessment of the role that ischemia plays in the diabetic foot requires a clinical examination and the use of noninvasive testing.

Clinical Evaluation. Inspection of an ischemic limb reveals skin pallor more pronounced on elevation, hair loss, and increased thickness of the nails. Dependent rubor will be present in advanced stages of ischemia. Upon palpation, the foot may be cool to cold, and the absence of pedal pulses confirms the presence of arteriosclerotic occlusive disease.

Noninvasive Testing. The measurement of flow velocity with Doppler apparatus gives a more accurate assessment of peripheral perfusion. Because of incompressibility of the tibial vessels in diabetics, ankle pressure can be falsely elevated. A more accurate assessment is made by a recording of toe pressure. A normal toe/brachial index is 0.75; 0.25 represents severe occlusive disease. By calculating the toe/brachial index and measuring segmental pressure, the practitioner can evaluate the level of obstruction on the arterial tree between the femoral vessels and the digital arteries.

RADIOGRAPHIC FINDINGS

Differentiation must be made between non-infectious osseous alterations in the diabetic foot and osteomyelitis. It is crucial to note that using the radiograph as an isolated entity without an in-depth clinical evaluation may easily lead to misdiagnosis.

Osteolysis is a common noninfectious finding in the diabetic. Resorption of bone usually begins as a sharply defined lesion in the metatarsal or phalangeal region or both. The metatarsal shaft takes the appearance of a "pencil" or "candlestick" deformity. The remaining bone appears sclerotic, giving the lytic process a burned-out appearance. Acute osteomyelitis rarely shows areas of sclerosis. In addition, osteolysis does not exhibit the extensive periosteal elevation that is seen in osteomyelitis. There is minimal or no soft tissue inflammation, and the patient may be asymptomatic.

Osteoporosis, which is a diffuse loss of bone mineral content, is another finding in the diabetic foot. Clinically this is important since it may predispose the patient to fracture.

Neuropathic joint (Charcot joint) produces the classic picture of bone lysis with marked fragmentation and eburnation. The joint space is decreased, the articulating bone margins are irregular, and osteophytes and bone resorption may be seen. There may be a tendency toward disarticulation and dissolution of the joints and calcification in and around the involved joints. The foot becomes shorter and wider. The radiographic appearance of osteomyelitis is similar in both diabetic and nondiabetic patients. Characteristic changes include soft tissue swelling, osteolysis, periosteal reaction, and sequestrum formation (see Chapter 17).

Often the radiographic changes lag behind the clinical evidence; therefore, in addition to conventional radiograph, technetium 99m, gallium 67, and indium 111 scans used separately or together may assist in making an earlier diagnosis. These osseous changes may be accompanied by the presence of gas in the soft tissue, an end result of the metabolism of organisms such as *Escherichia coli, Acinobacter aerogenes,* Pseudomonas, and Klebsiella.

At the completion of the evaluation, one should be able to classify the diabetic patient with foot pathology into one of the following categories: neuropathic foot, ischemic foot, or combined ischemic and neuropathic foot with or without superinfection.

MANAGEMENT

Although this discussion concentrates on diabetic foot problems, such considerations must form a portion of the overall management plan for the diabetic. Clearly, other physiologic systems must be evaluated, particularly the patient's serum glucose. The keynote to the treatment of the diabetic foot is prevention. The pain associated with polyneuropathy can be managed initially with simple analgesics (e.g., aspirin, acetaminophen, mefenamic acid). If they fail, then oral imipramine 50 mg at bedtime with the dosage increased stepwise as necessary to 150 mg can be used as well as other drugs, including amitriptyline, chlorpromazine, carbamazepine, and phenytoin. It is essential to recognize that pain associated with diabetic neuropathy is either an exclusion diagnosis after ischemia has been ruled out or a chronic condition that will spontaneously resolve when hypoesthesia becomes the dominant feature in the clinical picture.

Ischemic ulcers in diabetics should be recognized by clinical examination, evaluated by preoperative angiography, and revascularized if anatomically and technically feasible. If no reconstructible distal vessel is detectable on angiography, a below-knee amputation is often unavoidable.

Neuropathic ulcers can be subdivided into mild, moderate, or severe, depending on the depth of the ulcer, the presence or absence of bone involvement, and the presence of associated cellulitis or abscess.

TABLE 1. *Principles of Management of Neuropathic Ulcers in Diabetes*

	Clinical Appearance	Treatment
Mild	Superficial No cellulitis No osteomyelitis	Rest Culture and sensitivity testing Antibiotics (oral) Orthotic appliances Careful follow-up
Moderate	Deep ulcer Osteomyelitis? 0–2 cm cellulitis	Admission to surgery Culture-specific antibiotics (intravenous) Surgical debridement Local dressings Amputation? Bypass? Orthotic appliances Careful follow-up
Severe	Deep ulcer Osteomyelitis Cellulitis >2 cm	Admission to surgery Culture-specific antibiotics (intravenous) Surgical debridement Local wound care Amputation? Bypass? Orthotic appliances Careful follow-up

Some essential guidelines should be adhered to in the treatment of neuropathic ulcers.

1. Nonweightbearing is mandatory.

2. Soaking the wound only macerates the tissue but does not debride the necrotic tissue and should be avoided.

3. Enzymatic debridement of the wound is not advisable because of the lack of predictive response to the agent.

4. Although dextran polymer (Debrisan) may help in cleaning the wound, a wet to dry dressing of dilute povidone-iodine solution changed twice daily is the safest and most effective method of wound care combined with thorough wound debridement.

5. The use of vasodilators should be abandoned.

6. Hemorrheologic agents (pentoxifylline) have a limited role to play in patients with claudication due to diabetes associated with chronic occlusive arterial disease. The agents have no scientifically proven use in the treatment of diabetic foot ulcers.

Diabetic ulcers are a limb-threatening complication of the disease and require a very aggressive approach in order to avoid the potential risk of limb loss. Early referral to foot specialists and vascular surgeons is necessary in order to limit progression of disease.

PREVENTION

Although the pathogenic complications of diabetes mellitus such as angiopathy and neuropathy cannot be prevented, the resultant ulcerations and infections can. The patient must take an active role in management and constant monitoring of the feet to decrease the risk of serious foot problems. Patient education is crucial, and a list should be provided as a constant reminder of dos and don'ts (see Appendix II at the end of the book).

The feet must be inspected daily for signs of erythema, cuts, scratches, abrasions, blisters, and the buildup of callus. A family member may need to assist if the patient's vision is inadequate. If any of the above are noticed or any other abnormality is seen, the patient should contact the doctor. Patients should not cut their own nails, corns, or calluses. The feet should be washed daily with a mild soap and dried carefully, especially between the toes. Daily lubrication with a nonperfumed, lanolin-based lotion helps to avoid dryness and fissuring. Sometimes an antifungal preparation may be needed if dryness and peeling are due to dermatophytosis, but this should be prescribed by the patient's physician. Thick, preferably wool, socks without seams should be worn. Shoes must be inspected daily for foreign objects. Reduction of abnormal forces by means of orthosis and proper shoe gear is mandatory in the foot at risk of developing ulcerations. One type of orthosis is an insole that is used mostly to redistribute the plantar weight forces acting on the metatarsal heads, the distal tips of the digits, and the other plantar bony prominences that have a tendency to build excessive hyperkeratotic tissue and eventually ulcerate. The orthotic can also be designed to add support to the longitudinal arch of the foot and to the greater and lesser tarsus, especially for those diabetics with Charcot changes. Another type of orthosis is the prescription foot orthotic. The advantage of this type of custom-fabricated orthotic is that it allows more biomechanical control of the entire foot. It is crucial to note that once the appropriate insert or orthotic is fabricated, certain precautions must be taken to avoid causing lesions on other areas of the foot. A break-in period and constant observation for irritation or other problems, especially in the neuropathic foot, are essential.

In addition to foot orthosis, the prevention of soft tissue damage from continuous or intermittent pressures can be achieved by the selection of proper shoe gear. An inappropriately fitted shoe (i.e., too tight) can cause increased pressure and resultant soft tissue breakdown at the site of irritation. A shoe that is too loose can increase friction as the foot slips, resulting in ulcerations at bony prominences. The diabetic should be made aware that new shoes should not be worn for more than 2 hours at a time, and after each usage the foot must be examined for areas of irritation. The use of orthopedic shoes or modifications greatly reduces the risk of ulceration. Extra-depth shoes give more room from heel to toe. The additional height in the inside of the shoe also provides more latitude in fitting the patient with orthosis. The high toe box is a shoe modification needed for patients with contracted digits to prevent dorsal and distal digital ulcerations. The bunion last shoe, with an increased medial width, prevents friction and ulceration over the medial eminence. Molded shoes have also been used to prevent or treat neuropathic ulcerations. These shoes, made from a cast of the patient's foot, ensure proper fit and redistribute the forces of weight bearing more evenly.

Some materials can also be used directly to alleviate pressure areas and disperse the weight-bearing pattern of the foot. These materials must be used cautiously in the diabetic, because certain adhesives may be deleterious to the skin of a diabetic; moreover, any device placed around the toes or foot must be placed loosely, if at all, to avoid strangulation of tissue and further serious complications. Proper shoes, insoles, and orthotic devices along with appropriate foot care and hygiene should serve as a adjunct to good diabetic control in preventing pedal ulcerations.

SEPSIS

Sepsis is the most dreaded complication that can occur in a diabetic foot. Often these patients will present to the emergency department in ketoacidosis with signs of systemic sepsis. A complete examination of the patient reveals a swollen foot draining pus from an ulceration on the plantar surface. The dorsal location of the swelling is often misleading since most of the pathology is originating from the sole of the foot. An unexplained loss of glucose control in any diabetic patient should prompt a thorough examination of the feet.

Bacteriology

Microbiologic studies are mandatory to guide the antimicrobial therapy accurately. The average number of isolates is 3.2 bacterial species per patient. Superficial swab cultures of the wound are often inaccurate in their results and should be replaced with specimen harvested from deep tissues.

The presence of multiple organisms as shown in Table 2 underlines the importance of broad-spectrum antibiotic coverage upon admission.

Treatment

The diabetic patient with a septic foot represents an absolute surgical emergency, and initial management must focus on correction of the systemic aspects of sepsis: correction of hypovolemia, control of hyperglycemia, correction of metabolic acidosis, use of broad-spectrum antibiotics, and control of cardiovascular instability. Within 8–12 hours, the patient should undergo surgical drainage of the purulent collection. If the foot is well perfused with present pedal pulses, then wide debridement of all infected tissue is necessary along with toe amputation if osteomyelitis is present. Secondary wound coverage is performed when all sepsis has been controlled and good granulation tissue appears in the wound. In the absence of pedal pulses and if the hind foot is ischemic, an open guillotine amputation may be needed above the malleoli.

The clinical situation that has been discussed represents the end stage of a neglected diabetic ulcer and can, in fact, occur after what is considered trivial trauma. Such neglect can lead to limb loss and an occasional mortality. One cannot overemphasize the need for prevention, which begins in the physician's office. Meticulous examination of the feet of diabetics, the use of orthotics, and early referral

TABLE 2. *Organisms Most Commonly Found in Foot Ulcers in Diabetic Patients*

Organism	Percent
Gram-negative, aerobic	
Proteus species	55
Escherichia coli	30
Klebsiella species	20
Pseudomonas aeruginosa	15
Gram-positive, aerobic	
Streptococcus fecalis	45
Staphylococcus aureus	35
Streptococci (non-group A or D)	35
Staphylococcus epidermidis	30
Gram-negative, anaerobic	
Bacteroides fragilis	45
Bacteroides melaninogenicus	35
Gram-positive, anaerobic	
Peptococcus species	80
Clostridium species	35
Propionibacterium species	25

to the appropriate specialist (podiatrist, vascular surgeon) compose part of the multidisciplinary approach that will help eradicate the axiom that says, "Every diabetic with an infected foot deserves an amputation."

BIBLIOGRAPHY

1. Bell DSH: Lower limb problems in diabetic patients. Postgrad Med 89:237–244, 1991.
2. Giurini JM, Curzan JS, Gibbons GW, Habershaw GM: Charcot's disease in diabetic patients. Postgrad Med 89:163–169, 1991.
3. Harrelsen JM: Management of the diabetic foot. Orthop Clin North Am 20:605–620, 1989.
4. Kaschak TJ, et al: Radiology of the diabetic foot. Clin Podiatr Med Surg 5:849–857, 1988.
5. Joseph WS, et al: Microbiology and antimicrobial therapy of diabetic foot infections. Clin Podiatr Med Surg 7:467–481, 1990.
6. Levin ME: On the evaluation, prevention, and treatment of diabetic foot lesions. J Diabetic Complications 3:211–219, 1989.
7. Pecoraro RE, Reiber GE, Burgess EM: Pathways to diabetic limb amputation: Basis for prevention. Diabetes Care 13:513–521, 1990.

Chapter 17

INFECTION

Gus Constantouris, D.P.M., R.Ph.,
and Michael P. DellaCorte, D.P.M.

The foot is predisposed to a variety of infections that reflect both functional and environmental factors. Stress to both the skin and subcutaneous structures causes blisters, hematomas, inflammation, and fissures that often progress to superficial and sometimes deep tissue infections. Exposure to the elements can cause breakdown of the skin, giving access to causative agents. Shoes and socks or stockings, functioning primarily for protection, produce a closed environment that deprives the foot of light and fresh air and generates moisture from increased heat production and perspiration. The cause of the infection may not always be obvious, and the classic signs of infection may be misleading. The differential diagnosis includes gout, stress fracture, infection (both bacterial and fungal), dermatitis, and arthritis. The use of a tuning fork that is tapped and then placed on the metatarsal heads can differentiate fracture from the other possibilities: A fracture produces pain, whereas an infection or other disorder causes only vibrations.

Under ideal circumstances (hospital, clinic, office), a complete blood count with differential, culture and sensitivity testing of the wound base, and a chemistry panel should be obtained. The antibiotic prescribed should be narrow spectrum and specific for the causative bacteria (as noted on the culture report). Practically speaking, such lab work may not be readily available to office-based practitioners, and the culture and sensitivity require 24–48 hours. Therefore, an educated guess for the choice of antibiotic is necessary. Table 1 gives an overview of typical organisms, and antibiotics and their spectrum of coverage.

Traditionally, penicillin (e.g., Pen-Vee K) has been the drug of choice; it is inexpensive and effective. However, penicillinase-producing bacteria (i.e., *Staphylococcus aureus*) require the use of synthetic penicillins, such as dicloxacillin or cloxacillin. Such agents are not very broad spectrum, and they are expensive. A broad-spectrum antibiotic, such as a cephalosporin (e.g., cephalexin, cefadroxil) is a reasonable alternative. Cephalexin, 500 mg given orally every 6 hours for 7–10 days has a spectrum of coverage consisting of *Staphylococcus aureus*, Streptococcus group A, Klebsiella, *Escherichia coli,* and Proteus. Cefadroxil has a similar spectrum, but dosage is 500 mg given twice daily or 1 gram daily. Ciprofloxacin is another broad-range oral antibiotic that covers *Pseudomonas aeruginosa* and methicillin-resistant *Staphylococcus aureus* (traditionally covered only by intravenous antibiotics). It can be used as a first-line drug if the above organisms are suspected or if the patient is allergic to penicillin. (There is a 5–10% cross sensitivity to cephalosporins in the penicillin-allergic patient.) Ciprofloxacin is well tolerated orally and comes in 250, 500, and 750 mg doses given twice daily for 5–7 days. Intravenous ciprofloxacin is reserved for more serious cases because of its expense. Once culture results are available, the antibiotic therapy is adjusted based on sensitivities. If the wound is improving clinically, the initial antibiotic is generally continued for 10 days. Intravenous antibiotics, along with hospitalization, are warranted if no clinical improvement is noted, if systemic symptoms and signs are noted, or if there is history of poorly controlled diabetes or peripheral vascular disease.

TABLE 1. *Antimicrobial Drugs of Choice*

Infecting Organism	Drug of Choice	Usual Adult Dose	Alternative
Gram-positive cocci			
Staphylococcus aureus or *epidermidis* (nonpenicillinase)	Penicillin G, V	V: 1-2 gm/day PO Q6h G: 2-20 million units IV Q4-6h	Cephalosporin, vancomycin, clindamycin
S. aureus or *epidermidis* (penicillinase) Methicillin resistant	Penicillinase-resistant penicillin (cloxacillin, dicloxacillin) Vancomycin with or without rifampin and/or gentamicin	2-4 gm/day PO Q6h 2-12 gm/day IV Q4-6h 1-2 gm/day IV Q6-12h	Cephalosporin, vancomycin, clindamycin, trimethoprim/sulfamethoxazole, ciprofloxacin, imipenem
Streptococcus anaerobius; groups A, B, C, G; *bovis; milleri; pneumoniae;* or *viridans*	Penicillin G, V	As above	Cephalosporin, vancomycin, clindamycin, erythromycin
Streptococcus group D, enterococcus	Ampicillin Amoxicillin	2-8 gm/day IV Q4-6h 1-2 gm/day PO Q6h 0.75-2 gm/day PO Q6-8h	Vancomycin, imipenem, penicillin, aminoglycoside
Gram-positive bacilli			
Bacillus anthracis	Penicillin G, V	As above	Erythromycin, tetracycline, penicillin G, trimethoprim/sulfamethoxazole
Cornybacterium spout species	Erythromycin and antitoxin	1-4 gm/day IV Q6h	
Listeria monocytogenes	Ampicillin and gentamicin	1-2 gm/day PO Q6h	
Gram-negative cocci			
Neisseria meningitidis	Penicillin G	As above	Chloramphenicol, erythromycin, spectinomycin, tetracycline, cefoxitin, ampicillin
Neisseria gonorrhoeae	Penicillin G	As above	
Gram-negative bacilli			
Escherichia coli	Aminoglycoside (gentamicin) Cephalosporin	3-5 mg/kg/day IV or IM Q8h 250-500 mg PO QID	Ampicillin, trimethoprim/sulfamethoxazole, imipenem, aztreonam, oxacillin, ciprofloxacin, norfloxacin
Klebsiella	Cephalosporin with or without aminoglycoside	As above	Aminoglycoside, trimethoprim/sulfamethoxazole, piperacillin, mezlocillin, imipenem, ticarcillin, clavulanate, aztreonam, ciprofloxacin, norfloxacin, amoxicillin-clavulanate
Morganella morganii	Aminoglycoside Ciprofloxacin/norfloxacin	3-5 mg/kg/day IV or IM Q8h 750 mg PO BID	Imipenem, aztreonam, tetracycline, antipseudomonal penicillin, ticarcillin, amoxicillin, clavulanate
Enterobacter aerogenes or *cloacae*	Aminoglycoside Cephalosporin—third generation	As above	Aztreonam, imipenem, trimethoprim/sulfamethoxazole, antipseudomonal penicillin, ciprofloxacin
Citrobacter freundii	Imipenem, trimethoprim/sulfamethoxazole, aminoglycoside, ciprofloxacin, norfloxacin	1-4 gm/day IV Q6h	Tetracycline, cephalosporin—third generation
Pseudomonas aeruginosa	Aminoglycoside (gentamicin) Antipseudomonal penicillin (carbenicillin)	3-5 mg/kg/day IV or IM Q8h 8-40 gm/day IV Q4-6h	Aminoglycoside, cefoperazone, imipenem, ceftazidime, aztreonam, ciprofloxacin
Pseudomonas cepacia	Trimethoprim/sulfamethoxazole	2-20 mg/kg/day PO or IV Q6-8h	Chloramphenicol, ceftazidime
Pseudomonas mallei	Streptomycin and tetracycline	1-2 gm/day IM	Chloramphenicol, streptomycin
Pseudomonas maltophilia	Trimethoprim/sulfamethoxazole	2-20 mg/kg/day PO or IV Q6-8h	Ticarcillin-clavulanate
Proteus mirabilis	Ampicillin	2-8 gm/day IV Q4-6h 1-2 gm/day PO Q6h	Aminoglycoside, trimethoprim/sulfamethoxazole, aztreonam, imipenem, ciprofloxacin, antipseudomonal penicillin, cephalosporin—third generation
Proteus vulgaris	Cephalosporins—third generation (cefoperazone) Aminoglycoside	2-8 gm/day IM or IV Q8-12h As above	Trimethoprim/sulfamethoxazole, aztreonam, oxacillin, imipenem, amoxicillin, ticarcillin, clavulanate, ciprofloxacin

Table continued on next page.

TABLE 1. *Antimicrobial Drugs of Choice (Continued)*

Infecting Organism	Drug of Choice	Usual Adult Dose	Alternative
Gram-negative bacilli *(Cont.)*			
Pasteurella multocida	Penicillin G	2–20 million units IV Q4–6h	Tetracycline, erythromycin, cephalosporin, ampicillin
Haemophilus influenzae	Cephalosporin third generation (cefoperazone)	2–8 gm/day IM or IV Q8–12h	Chloramphenicol
	Trimethoprim/sulfamethoxazole	As above	
Anaerobes			
Bacteriodes fragilis group	Metronidazole	0.75–2 gm/day PO Q12h	Cefotetan, chloramphenicol,
	Clindamycin, cefoxitin, imipenem, ticarcillin	0.75–2 gm/day IV Q6–12h 1.8–2.7 gm/day IV Q6–8h	oxacillin, ampicillin, sulbactam
	Clavulanate	0.6–1.8 gm/day PO Q12h	
Clostridium species	Penicillin G	As above	Chloramphenicol, metronidazole, erythromycin, clindamycin, oxacillin, penicillin
Clostridium difficile	Vancomycin (oral)	0.5 gm–2.0 gm/day PO Q6h	Bacitracin (oral), cholestyramine
	Metronidazole (oral)	0.75–2.0 gm/day PO Q12h	
Peptostreptococcus	Penicillin G	2–20 million units IV Q4–6h	Clindamycin, metronidazole, cephalosporin, chloramphenicol, erythromycin, vancomycin, imipenem
Actinomyces israelii	Pencillin G	2–20 million units IV Q4–6h	Clindamycin, tetracycline, erythromycin

(BID = two times daily; h = hours; IM = intramuscularly; IV = intravenously; PO = orally; Q = every; QID = four times daily)

SPECIFIC INFECTIONS

Cellulitis

Cellulitis is an acute, severe, rapidly spreading skin infection. Lymphadenitis is an inflammatory swelling of regional lymph nodes recognizable by palpable, tender lymph nodes. The two most common agents causing cellulitis or lymphadenitis are group A *Streptococcus pyogenes* and *Staphylococcus aureus*. The severity of the disease is variable but warrants rapid diagnosis and treatment. Clinical presentation is characterized by hyperemia, edema, pain, increased local temperature, and decreased function. The causative microorganism and its by-products can travel proximally along anatomic pathways (e.g., subcutaneous tissue spaces, tendon sheaths, fascial spaces, muscles, lymphatics, and bone). The result may be bacteremia or septicemia. Both erythema and interdigital fungi with maceration can mimic a cellulitis. The diagnosis is sometimes difficult in these cases.

Although bacterial infections can result in a more disabling, painful infection, fungal infections are more prevalent in the foot. Combination infections (bacterial and fungal) are not uncommon. The differential diagnosis is determined clinically by noting the extent of the erythema, edema, and pain in the area. Extension proximal to the web space usually indicates cellulitis. Along with cellulitis, open portals and frank pus are diagnostic of infection. The macerated tissue interdigitally may appear as pus; therefore, debridement with a dry gauze prior to making the diagnosis is helpful. Bacterial cultures of any expressed material or drainage taken with a culturette should be sent for culture and sensitivity. Fungal cultures of the surrounding skin are not essential, although they serve to identify the presence of complicating fungal infections. The tinea should be managed with cotton socks and topical creams for 4–6 weeks. Creams and solutions promote drying; ointments macerate and should never be used in the interspace.

Unguis Incurvatus

The infected ingrown nail is a common occurrence in practice and, because of patient fear and ignorance, is not generally seen until the infection is severe. Generally, treating these wounds with antibiotics as a first course never completely heals the infection. The cause of the infection is a piece of toenail that penetrates into the skin and acts as a foreign body. The infection does not resolve until the offending nail is removed. Surgical matricectomy may be necessary in recurrent cases.

Infected Blister

Blisters result from constant friction or stress in one area of the foot. The pain that accompanies the blister formation usually forces the patient to change gait pattern or rest the feet. In cases in which the stress or friction is not removed or relieved, the blister usually opens, exposing the underlying raw base to bacteria. Localized painful infection results. In addition to management of the infection, treatment consists of debridement, dispersion padding, and warm water soaks or compresses.

Infected Fissures

Fissures are cracks in the skin that can be caused by fungus, dry skin conditions (e.g., xerosis), biomechanical abnormalities, or long-standing tylomata. Left untreated, the fissure progresses through the skin and into the subcutaneous tissue, causing pain and infection. Once infected, progression to cellulitis is rapid, so aggressive treatment is necessary. In addition to management of the infection, treatment consists of debridement of the fissure with a scalpel or tissue nipper to remove any hyperkeratotic or necrotic tissue. Dispersion padding and modifications in shoe gear may be necessary to relieve pressure. Modifications include cutting the shoe to relieve pressure and/or padding inside the shoe. Weekly debridements may be necessary until the condition resolves completely. If the etiology is biomechanical, foot orthotics may be indicated to prevent future infections.

Infected Laceration

The clinician should obtain a history of how and when the laceration occurred, along with any pertinent medical history (i.e., medications, diabetes, peripheral vascular disease). The patient should be questions for constitutional symptoms (e.g., fever, general malaise, chills) and tetanus immunization status. Vital signs are recorded, and the wound carefully inspected, measured, and palpated. A drawing of the wound should be noted in the chart. Treatment consists of rest, elevation, heat, debridement, lavage, and a broad-spectrum antibiotic. A dosage of 0.5 ml of tetanus toxoid should be administered intramuscularly according to the guidelines in

Chapter 13. Warm water soaks in Burow's solution or epsom salt may be effective in draining open wounds. Dry, sterile dressings should be applied to the wound after the soaks. Elevation above heart level has been the standard of care for allowing an edematous area to drain. In cases in which the pedal circulation is marginal, leaving the foot level relative to the heart increases tissue perfusion and antibiotic blood levels. The wound should not be sutured; secondary closure or delayed primary closure is the usual treatment.

OSTEOMYELITIS

The four main pathogenetic classifications of osteomyelitis are:

1. hematogenous—the spread of bacteria via the blood stream,

2. contiguous—the spread of infection from adjacent soft tissue to underlying bone, also known as secondary osteomyelitis,

3. direct inoculation—secondary to trauma or surgery, and

4. vascular insufficiency—caused generally by poor tissue perfusion

1. Hematogenous Osteomyelitis. The presence of pathogenic bacteria and other factors such as vascular stasus and a favorable bacterial growth medium (blood clot or necrotic tissue) are required. The vasculature at the level of the metaphysis in growing bone involves many hairpin turns and areas where blood flow is sluggish. Once a bacterial embolus reaches this level, sluggish blood flow may allow the embolus to settle in the periphery and cause thrombosis.

Retrograde occlusion, transudation, and necrosis of the marrow follow, producing a good environment for bacterial growth and colonization. This form of osteomyelitis is generally seen in the pediatric patient but can be noted in any age group. Surgical procedures on the foot, utilizing deep sutures, joint implants, buried wires, or screws, may also create a good environment for bacterial attachment and growth. The symptoms are usually pain and swelling, with possible alteration in gait pattern.

Treatment involves isolating the causative bacteria by either blood cultures, aspiration of the affected area, or both, followed by antibiotic therapy. Intensive intravenous antibiotics are necessary for 4–6 weeks in acute osteomyelitis; chronic cases may require longer therapy. Surgical intervention may also be necessary. Infectious disease and surgical consultations are in order.

2. Contiguous Osteomyelitis. This form of osteomyelitis is quite common in the diabetic with impaired sensation and circulation (Chapter 16). Long-standing ulcerations become infected and progress to bone. Other possible etiologies include abscesses, abrasions of the skin, long-standing paronychia, infected burns, and infected puncture wounds, with or without foreign bodies. The initial clinical presentation may vary depending on the causative factor and the patient's age, vascular status, and general health. Progressive pain, erythema, edema, and increased temperature in the affected area are the usual signs. Changes in gait and limping may evolve in order to avoid movement of the affected area.

3. Direct Inoculation. These cases are generally surgical. The bone is infected first, with later involvement of the soft tissue. Once the infection reaches the surface, the classic signs of infection may be masked by normal postoperative wound response. Diagnosis and treatment may, therefore, be delayed, causing a catastrophic outcome. Aseptic and sterile techniques, along with the use of prophylactic antibiotics in high-risk cases, constitute the best method of reducing this type of osteomyelitis.

4. Vascular Insufficiency. Decrease in blood flow to bone leads to stagnation and decreased oxygenation, creating an environment conducive to bacterial growth. The progression of the infection is slower because of poor tissue perfusion, and some of the classic signs, such as edema and increased temperature, may not be seen. Treatment with intravenous antibiotics is less effective due to poor tissue perfusion. Vascular surgery is often indicated to increase blood flow to the area.

Laboratory Tests

If osteomyelitis is suspected, a complete blood count, erythrocyte sedimentation rate (ESR), and blood cultures should be taken. The ESR is generally elevated. The initial white cell count may be normal, but the differential leukocyte count shows an increase in polymorphonuclear leukocytes. Any open sites or abscesses should be cultured. Both soft tissue and bone cultures for aerobic and anaerobic bacteria and fungus should be

taken in the hospital setting, prior to infusion of antibiotics. Gram stains should also be done on any drainage. A percutaneous bone biopsy and culture through a separate incision ensure against soft tissue contamination of the specimen. If a septic joint is involved, aspiration may be necessary.

X-ray Findings

Conventional x-rays generally do not show any signs of osteomyelitis for the first 10–14 days of infection. Areas of radiolucency caused by bone lysis may be the first radiographic signs (10–14 days). Periosteal lifting—Codman's triangle—which causes new bone formation, is a classic sign of osteomyelitis (14–21 days). The chronic phase of osteomyelitis is noted by the formation of sequestrae—highly opaque, smooth islands of bone that are usually surrounded by areas of decreased density termed involucra (21–28 days). As the infection progresses, a lytic tract through the cloaca may be variably seen (21–28 days).

There is no exact time sequence for these radiographic changes, although once noted, aggressive surgical treatment is warranted. X-rays of the noninfected foot and/or previous x-ray evaluation (if available) of the involved foot, compared with the most recent films, may show changes indicative of osteomyelitis.

When the diagnosis is suspected but not confirmed on conventional x-rays, a triphasic bone scan may be indicated. A technetium bone scan shows increased areas of uptake or "hot spots" in the infected bone, reflecting increased blood flow and increased bone turnover in an area. The scan is very sensitive but not too specific, since tumors, arthritis, and other inflammatory processes produce false-positives. The scan must be interpreted in light of both the clinical picture and the laboratory findings.

Treatment

Hospital admission is mandatory. Wound cultures and blood cultures should be taken prior to the start of antibiotic therapy. Medical conditions affecting the foot infection, such as diabetes and peripheral vascular disease, should be managed in conjunction with a specialist. If a definitive diagnosis of osteomyelitis cannot be established by x-ray or bone scan, a bone culture is advised. If the patient is on antibiotics, the medications should be discontinued for 48 hours prior to the bone culture. The culture should be taken from a site other than the ulcerated or infected area. A percutaneous specimen of bone should be analyzed pathologically as well as cultured aerobically, anaerobically, and fungally. Intravenous therapy alone for the "cure" of osteomyelitis can take months. The medications and dosages utilized vary, depending on the organisms isolated. The use of double and triple antibiotics is common. Once the diagnosis is made in the foot, the infected bone is surgically removed along with any infected tendon, capsule, and so on. The wounds are left open for local wound care and allowed to granulate. Skin grafting may be necessary, and amputation is not uncommon in these cases.

Often the defect left by the surgery takes longer to heal than the infection. Weekly in-office debridements and inspection of the wounds are necessary along with fabrication of orthotics or molded shoes to accommodate for defects.

BIBLIOGRAPHY

1. Arden S: The pathology of osteomyelitis. J Am Podiatr Med Assoc 67:702–705, 1977.
2. Axler DA, Terleckyj B, Abramson C: The microbiologic aspects of osteomyelitis. J Am Podiatr Assoc 67:691–699, 1977.
3. Donohue TW, Kanat IO: Radionuclides: Their use in osteomyelitis. J Am Podiatr Med Assoc 77:284–289, 1987.
4. Green NE, Edwards K: Bone and joint infections in children. Orthop Clin North Am 18:555–576, 1987.
5. Hill HG, Pitkow HS, Davis RH: The pathophysiology of osteomyelitis. J Am Podiatr Med Assoc 67:687–690, 1977.
6. Jahss MH (ed): Disorders of the Foot, Vol. II. Philadelphia, W.B. Saunders, 1982, pp 1398–1428.
7. Karlin JM: Osteomyelitis in children. Clin Podiatr Surg 4:37–56, 1987.

Chapter 18

VASCULAR PROBLEMS

Daniel L. Picard, M.D.

Atherosclerosis is a generalized and debilitating disease with protean manifestations. It frequently affects the lower extremities, with symptoms ranging from intermittent claudication to frank gangrene that results in limb loss. Over 100,000 vascular reconstructive procedures in the lower extremities are performed annually in the United States. Although the surgical results are good, the long-term survival of patients is, on average, 50% at 5 years, illustrating the generalized and severe nature of atherosclerosis.

PATHOPHYSIOLOGY

In order to offer any rational therapeutic plan for treatment of patients with atherosclerosis, clinicians must be familiar with the pathophysiology of the disease. Large epidemiologic studies have enabled the medical profession to identify specific risk factors associated with atherosclerosis. The major factors are hypertension, hypercholesterolemia, and cigarette smoking. The remaining minor risk factors have a more variable correlation with atherosclerosis but cannot be separated as independent predictors of the disease: obesity, diabetes mellitus, hypertriglyceridemia, sedentary living, stress, and family history. The pathologic changes associated with atherosclerosis are well-known and affect the three different layers that make up the arterial wall. The tunica media and intima are affected primarily, resulting in raised and ulcerated plaques and thrombosis.

Tissue proliferation is characteristic of all lesions, as are increased amounts of collagen and ground substance. Both intracellular and extracellular lipid infiltration are hallmarks of atherosclerosis. Finally, tissue reaction adjacent to areas of atherosclerosis is seen with platelet buildup and infiltration of inflammatory cells in the periplaque area. Atherosclerosis generally becomes symptomatic by progressive occlusion of the blood supply to the involved extremity or organ. Pain at the outset followed in time by tissue compromise occurs when the cross-sectional lumen of the vessel is reduced by 75%.

CLINICAL EVALUATION

History

Pain is the most common presenting symptom in patients with peripheral vascular disease. The pain's distinctive character, location, duration, and precipitating and relieving factors are elicited and allow the diagnosis of arterial disease to be made in 90% of the cases. Intermittent claudication is frequently described as tiredness or a cramp when walking; it is relieved by rest. Its location is related to the site of critical stenosis. Aortoiliac occlusive disease manifests itself in the buttocks and thighs; a superficial femoral artery occlusion typically presents itself with calf claudication.

Pain at rest is present when the affected limb is threatened by gangrene. It is a surgical emergency requiring vascular surgical evaluation and hospitalization. The review of symptoms focuses on the generalized nature of the atherosclerosis. Signs of cerebrovascular insufficiency are noted: transient ischemic attacks, amaurosis fugax, transient aphasia, and dizziness. Likewise, the practitioner should interrogate the patient regarding past cardiac history while searching for symptoms of ischemic heart disease. Finally, both major and minor risk factors should be identified. The physical examination includes heart rate and rhythm, bilateral blood pressure measurement, neck auscultation for carotid bruits, cardiac auscultation, abdominal palpation to search for aneurysms, abdominal auscultation for bruits, palpation of peripheral pulses, auscultation of groins and femoral areas for bruits, and inspection of the legs and feet for ulcers and gangrene. A systematic examination of the lower extremities yields considerable information that confirms the suspected diagnosis. Inspection, palpation, and auscultation reveal the chronic and acute changes associated with arterial insufficiency.

Early chronic disease does not appreciably change the appearance of the leg. Hair loss is not a consistent sign of arterial insufficiency. Muscle atrophy may appear later in the course of the disease. Dependent rubor of the forefoot is one of the most reliable indicators of severe ischemia; it is followed by tissue necrosis (i.e., ulcers or gangrene if no treatment is rendered). Commonly, the ulcers are small in size, shallow with irregular edges, and located distally on the foot or the anterior aspect of the leg. No evidence of granulation tissue confirms the ischemic nature of these ulcers. Venous ulcers, by comparison, are located in the territory of the draining veins (i.e., the greater saphenous vein). Above the medial malleolus, they are large, usually indolent, and associated with stasis dermatitis and varicose veins. Good granulation tissue is visible in the bed of the ulcer.

Acute arterial ischemia produces visible skin changes: pallor initially, followed in time by mottling. Within 24 hours of complete ischemia, the extremity becomes swollen with blisters. Gangrenous changes may take days to appear. Comparative palpation of the extremity assesses the lower-extremity temperature against that of the upper limbs.

Palpation of pulses is a critical step in the assessment of the patient and should be graded. A simple system notes the presence or absence of pulses. A more subjective method is to grade on a scale of 1 to 4 the quality of the pulse:

0, absent
1+, barely palpable
2+, diminished
3+, normal
4+, prominent and possibly associated with aneurysmal dilatation

The femoral pulse lies below the inguinal ligament, two finger-breadths lateral to the pubic tubercle. The popliteal pulse is often difficult to palpate and requires that the patient be in a supine position, with the knee partially flexed, resting on one of the examiner's hands, while the other sinks gently into the popliteal space. The posterior tibial pulse is located behind the medial malleolus; the dorsalis pedis artery is palpable on the dorsum of the foot between the first and the second metatarsal bones. The absence of the dorsalis pedis pulse may be a congenital variant in 10% of cases. Auscultation of the abdomen and the femoral area may reveal bruits indicative of occlusive disease of the aorta or the iliac arteries. Finally, a neurologic examination is indispensable to assess epicritic sensation, muscle strength, and presence or absence of deep tendon reflexes. At the completion of the physical examination, the physician is able to recognize one of three clinical pictures.

1. Intermittent claudication represents a stage of non-limb-threatening ischemia.

2. Threatened limb loss is associated with rest pain, dependent rubor, nonhealing ulcer, or frank gangrenous changes.

3. Acute arterial ischemia is commonly referred to as the **three Ps:** pain, pallor, and pulselessness at an early stage. If progression ensues, two additional Ps appear: paresthesias and paralysis.

Differential Diagnosis

Pain of hip arthritis and sciatica is fairly characteristic but may mimic claudication and hence is referred to as pseudoclaudication syndrome. Normal pedal pulses associated with classic musculoskeletal and neurologic findings establish the diagnosis. Diabetic neuropathy may be too subtle to recognize at an early stage. A more complete description of this condition is found in Chapter 16. Reflex sympathetic dystrophy or minor causalgia produces a burning pain, but the presence of normal peripheral pulses supports the diagnosis.

VASCULAR LABORATORY STUDIES

Although noninvasive tests have been a useful adjunct in assessing the patient with peripheral vascular disease, they do not replace a thorough history and physical examination. The instrumentation should be simple, reliable, and reproducible. Adaptability to recording devices is highly desirable for record-keeping and comparison. The two most useful instruments available are the continuous-wave Doppler system and the pulse volume recorder, or segmental plethysmograph.

More recently, technologic advances have made use of real-time ultrasound (also called B mode ultrasound) as a reliable tool to investigate the arterial and venous systems.

In office practice, the Doppler probe suffices to examine all major peripheral arteries with great accuracy. A Doppler survey includes the acoustic assessment of both ankle arteries (dorsalis pedis and posterior tibial). A normal arterial signal has two or sometimes three components. The first part is a high-pitched sound that represents forward flow during systole. A brief lower-pitched sound represents the second component and corresponds to the reversal flow in early diastole. A third low-pitched sound may be heard as the forward flow resumes. The presence or absence of sound at the ankle should be noted at the time of initial survey. The presence of a monophasic sound indicates proximal stenosis or occlusion. Objective recording is then made of the absolute ankle pressure and compared with the systemic arm pressure. The ankle/brachial ratio or index (ABI) should be equal to or greater than 1.0. An index of 0.75 is usually associated with claudication, whereas a value of 0.5 or less reflects severe limb-threatening ischemia.

Segmental leg pressures can be misleading in diabetics with severely calcified vessels that are not compressible. In these patients, normal or abnormally high pressure readings can be recorded even though severe ischemic changes are taking place in the foot.

ANGIOGRAPHY

Angiography is indicated for patients who are candidates for vascular reconstruction. It should be emphasized that angiography is an invasive test that is mandatory for preoperative mapping, but it is not a diagnostic modality.

Technique. Angiography is more commonly performed via the transfemoral route using the Seldinger technique. The translumbar or transaxillary approaches are available if the femoral route is impractical. Angiography requires an arterial puncture. Digital subtraction technique has more recently been introduced, which makes use of computer image reconstruction to enhance the quality of the radiographs.

It can also be used via the transvenous route. The complications of angiography include bleeding from arterial puncture. Allergic reactions to the contrast medium and renal failure can be reduced by the use of noniodinated dye.

Mortality related to angiography is a rare event (0.05%) but a definite risk that the patient should understand. It is probable that magnetic resonance angiography will soon be available to obtain vascular imaging without any injection of contrast medium, thus reducing the risks for the patient.

Results. Atherosclerotic occlusive disease is defined as being located above or below the inguinal ligament. Above the inguinal ligament, the distal abdominal aorta and the iliac bifurcation are the most common sites of pathology and such disease is referred to as aortoiliac occlusive disease. Because it impedes flow to the lower extremities below the groin, it is also referred to as inflow disease. Below the inguinal ligament, the most common site of arterial occlusive disease is the superficial femoral artery at Hunter's canal. The distal arteries can also be affected, namely, the popliteal artery or its most distal branches, the anterior tibial, posterior tibial, and peroneal arteries. These vessels are more commonly affected in diabetics. Arterial occlusive disease below the knee is referred to as outflow disease.

Only once the angiogram is completed does the vascular surgeon become able to recommend the appropriate therapeutic modality to the patient.

PREVENTION

Cessation of smoking is essential but often difficult to achieve. Control of hypertension and hyperglycemia is necessary and may have to be achieved urgently if surgery is necessary for limb salvage. Normalizing the lipid profile of a patient is likely to be beneficial on a long-term basis but is more of a preventive modality than a curative one in the face of established and symptomatic atherosclerosis. Regular aerobic exercise and weight reduction are also desirable for their systemic benefits.

THERAPY

Medical Treatment

The therapeutic approach by the practitioner for a patient presenting with lower-extremity ischemia is multidisciplinary, targeting both the systemic and focal aspects of the disease. Medical therapy is aimed at both controlling the risk factors that contribute to atherosclerosis and, in a more limited way, attempting to alleviate the consequences of arterial ischemia.

A variety of medications have been attempted in treating patients with symptomatic peripheral vascular disease. Vasodilators are not recommended. Similarly, oral anticoagulants have no proven use in the treatment of a patient with symptomatic peripheral vascular disease. Warfarin treatment is indicated and is effective in the prevention of embolic phenomena in the lower extremities. Platelet antiaggregants (dipyridamole, 25 mg three times daily, or acetylsalicylic acid, 325 mg every day) play a limited prophylactic role in the postoperative stage after vascular reconstruction but are not effective in a patient with intermittent claudication.

Unconventional therapies such as intravenous chelating agents or megavitamins have no proven effect in reversing the ravages of atherosclerosis on the arterial wall.

The hemorrheologic agent pentoxifylline modifies the deformability of erythrocytes and has emerged as the only medication with some proven, albeit limited, efficacy in the treatment of intermittent claudication. Administered at the dose of 400 mg three times daily, one might expect some improvement in the patient's symptoms after 8 weeks of therapy. However, it has no proven clinical efficacy in patients with limb-threatening ischemia (i.e., ischemic ulcerations or gangrene). All patients who present with symptoms of intermittent claudication should be started on a controlled exercise program aimed at improving distance tolerance. Claudication in itself is relatively benign, since only 10% of patients incur limb loss after 5 years.

Surgical Treatment

Surgery is indicated for limb salvage only in patients with evidence of rapidly progressive claudication or limb-threatening ischemia with rest pain, ischemic ulcers, or frank gangrene.

Open Vascular Reconstruction. Vascular surgery has proved to be extremely effective and durable in achieving limb salvage. Aortoiliac occlusive disease can be corrected by endarterectomy or bypass technique. The 5-year patency of the reconstruction is about 85%. An extra-anatomical bypass (axillofemoral or femorofemoral bypass) might be indicated for high-risk patients and also achieve good results. These procedures are aimed at correcting inflow disease. Disease of the femoropopliteal axis may be reconstructed using femoropopliteal or femorotibial bypasses. Autogenous saphenous vein reversed or in situ is the most desirable conduit for reconstruction. Synthetic material is also available for bypass. The 5-year patency rate of autogenous saphenous vein graft is 68%, compared with 38% for synthetic grafts. The overall limb salvage rate at 5 years is in excess of 70% with vein grafts.

Angioplasty. Percutaneous balloon angioplasty is an accepted reconstruction technique that has proved to be effective and durable in the iliac vessels. A 5-year patency rate of 85% can be expected. Angioplasty has the advantage of being relatively noninvasive, and failure does not preclude the surgeon from performing a conventional open bypass. The recent adjunct of laser technology to assist in the performance of balloon angioplasty is generating interest in treating occlusion of the superficial femoral or popliteal artery. At present, patencies of 70% are being reported at 3–6 months after performance of the procedure. No long-term results are yet available.

Arterial Embolectomy. Thromboembolectomy of fresh thrombus of the iliac or the femoral artery can be successful in patients who present with signs of acute arterial ischemia. Thrombolytic agents (streptokinase, urokinase, tissue plasminogen activator) may be effective when used as sole therapeutic agents or in conjunction with embolectomy catheters. The overall limb salvage rate averages 85% in patients suffering from acute ischemia secondary to arterial embolism.

Lumbar Sympathectomy. Popularized by Rene Leriche before bypasses were available, the role of lumbar sympathectomy is currently limited to patients suffering from causalgia and vasospastic diseases. It is occasionally used in patients with small ischemic foot ulcerations who have no vessels suitable for vascular reconstruction.

Amputation. Lower-extremity amputation is often the end point of peripheral vascular disease. It is necessary to perform amputation either to control sepsis originating from the lower extremity or in the face of established gangrene. The therapeutic goals are primary wound healing and rehabilitation so that the patient can walk again. Selecting a proper amputation level is based on clinical evaluation and knowledge of the disease extent in an individual patient. The different levels range from single-digit ablation to transmetatarsal amputation. These are associated with excellent functional results. Below-knee and above-knee amputations are much more debilitating, especially among the elderly population, in whom peripheral vascular disease is common. Although perioperative mortality averages 10% in major amputations, long-term survival is poor, with a 50% mortality in the 3 years following surgery. Of the survivors, a third to a half require a contralateral amputation within 3 years.

BIBLIOGRAPHY

1. Brewster DC (ed): Common Problems in Vascular Surgery. Chicago, Year Book Medical Publishers, 1989, pp 231–236.
2. Ernst CB, Stanley JC (eds): Current Therapy in Vascular Surgery. Toronto, B.C. Decker, 1987, pp 193–247.
3. Kemczinski RF: The Ischemic Leg. Chicago, Year Book Medical Publishers, 1985.

Chapter 19

MISCELLANEOUS CONDITIONS

Richard B. Birrer, M.D.,
and Michael P. DellaCorte, D.P.M.

TUMORS

Malignant tumors of the foot are rare, and benign tumors and tumorlike lesions are uncommon (Table 1). However, deformities, swelling, and protuberances of a nontumorous etiology are quite common. Confusion of nontumorous lesions with tumorous ones often leads to delayed diagnosis and inappropriate conservative therapy.

Symptoms usually include swelling, pain, deformity, and dysfunction. The physical exam confirms the presentation, but laboratory tests (complete blood count; an automated chemistry panel, including calcium, immunoglobulins, and serum enzyme levels [phosphatases]; radiologic tomography and angiography; and radioisotopic scanning [technetium phosphate]), computerized tomography or magnetic resonance imaging studies, or both are usually required. Definitive diagnosis is made by a biopsy. The technique may be incisional, excisional, or by curettage and can be performed with a needle or by an open excisional approach. Whenever possible, the latter approach is preferred, because adequate tissue can be obtained and the risk of local and systemic contamination is minimized. Normal tissue must always be included in the sample. Consultation with a surgeon and oncologist is advised for all malignant and complex benign tumors.

NEUROLOGIC DISORDERS AFFECTING THE FOOT

Diagnosis of nervous disorders affecting the foot is difficult due to the complexity of the nervous system and the variable, often subtle manifestations of neurologic disease. These neurologic problems encompass a vast collection of complaints, symptoms, and etiologies (Table 2) for which referral to a neurologic specialist is essential in early podiatric management of such patients.

Clinical manifestations of neurologic disorders affecting the foot generally arise from the peripheral nervous system (Table 2). Central nervous system disease is often secondary to spinal cord compression, convulsions, stroke, and coma and is infrequently seen in the foot. Disorders of peripheral nerves may affect the foot in several ways, including paresis, paralysis, sensory defects, pain, and contractures. When these changes occur quickly, the patient usually notices and reports a change in function. However, when deficits develop slowly, the patient may ignore the reduced sensation or motor power. Pain resulting from peripheral neuropathy may be the most devastating symptom. Treatment often requires pharmacologic, physiotherapeutic, psychologic, and surgical intervention, especially in posttraumatic cases. Associated manifestations of peripheral neuropathies include calf weakness (from paralysis of the posterior tibial nerve) and foot drop or an equinus deformity (from peroneal nerve paralysis). The sympathetic nervous system should also be evaluated in patients with pain, with special reference to absence of sweating and poor response to hot and cold, indicating sympathetic degeneration.

Examination of the patient with suspected neurologic disease should include evaluation of sensation, strength, reflexes, coordination, and gait (see Chapter 2).

TABLE 1.   Foot Tumors

	Benign	Malignant
Tumors/lesions of skin	Nevi Viral lesions Keratosis Keratoacanthoma Eccrine poroma Epidermal inclusion cyst Keloids	Melanoma Verrucous carcinoma Squamus cell carcinoma Basal cell carcinoma Malignant sweat gland tumors
Tumors of fibrous tissue and of fat	Fibroma Nodular fasciitis Plantar fibromatosis Juvenile aponeurotic fibroma Lipoma	Fibrosarcoma Dermatofibroma protuberans Liposarcoma
Tumors of muscle, tendons and joints	Leiomyoma Rhabdomyoma Giant cell tumor of tendon sheath Ganglion cyst Digital mucous cyst	Leiomyosarcoma Rhabdomyosarcoma Malignant giant cell tumor Synovial sarcoma Clear cell sarcoma
Tumors and lesions of nerves	Neuroma Neurofibroma Neurilemmoma Myoblastoma	Malignant neurofibroma Malignant neurilemmoma Malignant schwannoma
Tumors and lesions of blood vessels	Capillary hemangioma Cavernous hemangioma Venous hemangioma Hemangiopericytoma Glomus	Angiosarcoma Malignant hemangiopericytoma
Tumors and lesions of cartilage	Chondroblastoma Chondromyxoid fibroma Enchondroma Juxtacortical chondroma Osteochondroma	Chondrosarcoma Myxosarcoma
Tumors and lesions of bone marrow		Myeloma Ewing's sarcoma Reticular cell sarcoma Malignant lymphoma
Tumors and lesions of bone	Osteoma Osteoblastoma Osteoid osteoma	Osteosarcoma Malignant osteoblastoma
Tumorlike lesions of bone	Solitary bone cyst Aneurysmal bone cyst Giant cell tumor Myositis ossificans Nonossifying fibroma Eosinophilic granuloma	

Adapted from Berlin SJ: Tumors and tumerous conditions of the foot. In McGlamry ED (ed): Comprehensive Textbook of Foot Surgery. Baltimore, Williams & Wilkins, 1987, pp 609–645.

ENTRAPMENT NEUROPATHIES

Tarsal tunnel syndrome is caused by entrapment of the posterior tibial nerve as it passes behind the medial malleolus. The entrapment can be caused by inflammatory collagen vascular diseases, tumors, varicosities, chronic flexor tenosynovitis, or chronic severe pronation. The most common cause is usually fibrosis related to trauma. Symptoms consist of a burning sharp pain or a paresthesia that radiates into the sole of the foot toward the toes. The symptoms are intermittent, but they increase with prolonged activity. Clinically, there is a positive Tinel's sign (e.g., percussion of the posterior tibial nerve at the level of the medial malleolus, causing paresthesias distal to the toes). Definitive diagnosis is made by nerve conduction velocities and electromyographic studies, and once it has been

TABLE 2.   *Clinical Manifestations of Neurologic Disorders Affecting the Foot*

Disorder	Area of Primary Pathology	Etiology	Pedal Manifestations
Hereditary peripheral neuropathies Charcot-Marie-Tooth	Peroneal muscle atrophy	Dominant or recessively inherited	Pes cavus Muscle wasting Paresis Steppage gait Drop foot deformity Decreased/absent ankle jerk and vibratory sensation
Dejerine-Sottas disease (hypertrophic interstitial polyneuropathy)	Enlargement of peripheral nerves (peroneal nerve)	Autosomal recessive mechanism	Pes cavus Foot drop Loss of tendon reflexes
Roussy-Levy syndrome	Peripheral nerves	Dominantly inherited	Essential tremor Clumsy gait Absent tendon reflexes Foot atrophy
Refsum's disease (heredopathia ataxia polyneuritiformis)	Nerves	Autosomal recessive	Progressive paralysis Drop foot Pes cavus Ankle reflexes
Friedreich's ataxia	Cerebellum Cord Peripheral nerve	Posterior and caudal spinal cord degeneration (recessively inherited)	Pes cavus Ataxia Drop foot Peroneal nerve paresis Lurching Trendelenburg gait Babinski response
Cerebral vascular accident (stroke)	Cerebrum Ischemia to brain, with infarction	Hemorrhage Thrombosis Embolism to brain	Spastic contractures Equinovarus Claw-toe deformity Spastic equinus deformity Drop foot Babinski response
Muscular dystrophy (Duchenne's)	Muscle fibers (dystrophism)	X-linked inherited	Ankle equinus Equinovarus Paresis Loss of reflexes Secondary contractures
Spinal cord abnormalities	Lumbar and sacral areas	Failure of neural arch to close during development	Depends on level and extent of involvement
Spina bifida with meningocele (meninges and sac protrude through defect), myelomeningocele (additional element of spinal cord and nerve root protrusion), or myelocele (most severe: skin failed to close over neural elements); spina bifida occulta (all neural elements remain in spinal canal)			Pes cavus Equinus Equinovarus Valgus deformities Mild neurological deficits (spina bifida occulta)
Poliomyelitis	Viral infection of anterior horn cells of spinal cord Paralysis of innervated muscle	Viral infection Destruction of anterior Horn cells (enterovirus)	Paralysis of tibialis anterior Permanent lower motor neuron paralysis with paralytic-type polio Muscle contracture Muscle wasting Limb length discrepancy
Cerebral palsy Types:	Lesions of:	Brain lesion Congenital neuromuscular disease	Ankle equinus Spastic equinus
Spastic (most common)	Frontal lobe	Congenital maldevelopment of brain	Flexion, adduction, internal rotation of hip, knee, genu valgum

Continued on next page.

TABLE 2.   *Clinical Manifestations of Neurologic Disorders Affecting the Foot (Cont.)*

Disorder	Area of Primary Pathology	Etiology	Pedal Manifestations
Cerebral palsy *(Cont.)* Types:	Lesions of:		
Athetoid	Basal ganglia	Cerebral anoxia during perinatal period	Scissors gait Secondary talipes equino-

Ataxic	Cerebellar and eighth cranial
	  nerve
		Trauma during
		  birth
			valgus
			Talipes calcaneus

Rigid	Basal ganglia		Pes cavus
Tremor	Basal ganglia and cerebellar		Hallux valgus
Dystonic	Combination of the above		Hammertoe deformities

Diabetic neuropathy	Peripheral nerves
	  (vasonervorum) and
	  (posterior column)
	Autonomic nerve neuropathy
		Hyperglycemia
		Metabolic changes
		Segmental
		  demyelination
		Loss of Schwann cells
			Stocking/glove distribution
			Sensation of pain, temperature,
			  and touch decreased
			Impaired proprioception
			Sluggish or absent deep-
			  tendon reflexes
			Denervation of intrinsic muscles
			Hammer toes
			Charcot joints
			Malperforans ulcers

Sciatica	Distribution of sciatic nerve	Sacralization of the
		  fifth lumbar vertebrae
		Arthritis of the inter-
		  articular joints
		Spondylitis
		Tumor, especially
		  cauda equina
		Infection
		Hernia
			Steppage gait
			Dorsiflexion of foot
			Increased pain (Bragardis sign)
			Flexion of great toe
			Increased pain (Sicardi's sign)
			Achilles reflex lost or decreased
			Pain on straight-leg raise
			  (Lasegue's sign)

Peripheral neuritis	Peripheral nerves	Alcohol
		Beriberi
		Arsenic
			Painful hyperesthesias
			  of the soles of feet
			Short, painful steps
			Gait has a limping, halting
			  character with the feet rotated
			  in such a position as to avoid
			  walking on the painful
			  portions

Cerebral arterio- sclerosis	Circle of Willis	Senility	Short-stepped shuffling gait

Parkinson's disease
  (paralysis agitans)
	Basal ganglia	Arteriosclerosis
		Encephalopathy
		Senility
			Loss of automatic swing
			  of arms
			Initiation of act of shuffling
			  is slow
			Gait is slow and shuffling

Dystonia musculorum	Basal ganglia	Idiopathic
		Infection
		  Vascular disease of
		  the brain
		  Toxic conditions
		  Tumors
			Gait is characterized by
			  severe contortions, giving
			  a ludicrous, bizarre
			  appearance to
			  the act

confirmed, treatment is geared toward severity of symptoms and etiology. Rest, strapping, and nonsteroidal anti-inflammatory drugs (NSAIDs) are indicated initially. Injection therapy and orthotic control of abnormal foot function are recommended thereafter. No more than six injections should be given. If conservative therapy fails, surgical intervention to decompress the nerve is indicated.

LATERAL PLANTAR (CALCANEAL) NERVE ENTRAPMENT

Approximately 10–15% of athletes with chronic unresolving heel pain have entrapment of the lateral plantar nerve between the deep fascia of the abductor hallucis muscle and the medial caudal margin of the quadratus plantae muscle. Although running and jogging are the major causes, soccer, tennis, dancing, and track and field events are also provocative. There is usually chronic heel pain (for 1-2 years) that is dull, aching, or sharp. The pain may radiate into the ankle and is intensified by walking or running. There is point tenderness over the first branch of the lateral plantar nerve deep to the abductor hallucis muscle. Tinel's sign is infrequently positive, and a hypermobile foot may be noted. While the patient is stretching, NSAIDs, injection therapy, and orthotics should be tried. Their variable success rates often lead to surgical neurolysis.

PERONEAL NERVE ENTRAPMENT

The deep peroneal nerve can be entrapped in several locations, most commonly under the inferior extensor retinaculum (anterior tarsal tunnel syndrome). The superficial peroneal nerve can be entrapped at its exit point from the deep fascia. Although acute trauma in the form of recurrent ankle sprains is the major culprit underlying these neuropathies, repetitive microtrauma from running, soccer, tennis, dancing, skiing, and hockey subjects the nerves to recurrent stretching. Deep peroneal involvement is suggested by dorsal foot pain that is dull, aching, sharp, or spasmodic and that may radiate to the first toe web. There are both decreased sensation in the first toe web and reproduction of the pain with either dorsiflexion or plantarflexion. Superficial neuropathy is suggested by pain, paresthesias, or numbness over the other border of the distal calf, foot, and ankle dorsum. There may be point tenderness and a fascial defect where the nerve emerges from the deep fascia. Activity worsens both conditions, and there is usually a history of recurrent sprains or trauma. Conservative modalities include NSAIDs, physical therapy, orthotics, and injection therapy. Neurolysis is reserved for cases of intractable pain and atrophy (deep peroneal neuropathy).

SURAL NERVE ENTRAPMENT

Running activities can lead to entrapment of the sural nerve anywhere along its course. There is usually a history of an acute twisting injury and recurrent ankle sprains. Shooting pain and paresthesias are typical and are confirmed by local tenderness, a positive Tinel's sign, and occasionally an area of hyperesthesias. A trial of NSAIDs, orthotics, physical therapy, and injection therapy should be tried, although surgical release is usually definitive.

MEDIAL PLANTAR (CALCANEAL) NERVE ENTRAPMENT— JOGGER'S/RUNNER'S FOOT

Entrapment of the medial calcaneal branch of the posterior tibial nerve causes acute irritation and inflammation as well as chronic fibrosis and neuroma formation. The patient, usually a runner, jogger, or avid walker, complains of aching pain along the medial border of the heel that is more severe on weight bearing but does not radiate further forward into the foot. A planovalgus deformity or hyperpronation of the foot tends to aggravate the condition further. Anti-inflammatory agents and custom-molded orthotics are good conservative therapies. If the patient does not respond to these modalities after several months, operative neurolysis should be considered.

BIBLIOGRAPHY

1. Campbell CJ: Tumors of the foot. In Jahss MH (ed): Disorders of the Foot, Vol. 1. Philadelphia, W.B. Saunders, 1982, pp 979-1013.
2. Schon LC, Baxter DE: Neuropathies of the foot and ankle in athletes. Clin Sports Med 9:489-510, 1990.
3. Schubiner JM, Simon MA: Primary bone tumors in children. Orthop Clin North Am 18:577-596, 1987.

Chapter 20

GENERAL TREATMENT GUIDELINES

Michael P. DellaCorte, D.P.M.

The goal of any treatment plan is to relieve symptoms and, if possible, to cure the illness. Unfortunately, many illnesses cannot be cured, so treatment plans must be structured to maximize function. The purpose of this chapter is to discuss the indications, contraindications, methodology, and outcome of common foot procedures and devices.

PARING

Indication: Temporary relief of pain associated with tyloma and heloma. The patient should be made aware of the underlying cause of the corn or callus and informed that paring is not a permanent treatment.

Contraindication: Severe peripheral vascular disease.

Procedure: Paring is a conservative, noninvasive technique done with a scalpel handle and blade. The novice may wish to start with a No. 15 or No. 10 blade that fits a No. 3 handle; the experienced practitioner uses a No. 20 scalpel blade along with a No. 4 handle. The scalpel blade should be sterile. The patient's feet should be elevated to a comfortable level; the practitioner should be seated. The nondominant hand supports the foot, while the other debrides the corn or callus (Figs. 1 and 2). The scalpel blade is held firmly between the thumb and index finer and positioned almost parallel to the lesion (Fig. 3). With a slicing, semicircular motion, superficial amounts of corn or callus are debrided repeatedly until healthy pink tissue is noted. For safety, the cutting edge of the scalpel is always moving away from the practitioner; digital corns require a backhand stroke to

accomplish this (Figs. 4A and B). After the superficial debridement of the corn is completed, the central core must be removed to relieve symptoms. This deeper core is removed with the tip of the scalpel blade in a circular manner (Fig. 4C). Care must be taken to avoid cutting into the underlying healthy tissue, which would cause more pain than the corn. The procedure is time-consuming, and rushing through it may cause unnecessary iatrogenic lesions. Inflamed bursae underlying a corn may warrant a local injection of lidocaine prior to debridement. Debridement of callus may uncover hidden corns, foreign bodies, or ulcerations. The treatment plan may have to be altered depending on the findings.

Outcome/Prognosis: Six to 8 weeks of relief from the pain associated with heloma and tyloma (at which time the process is repeated).

PADDING

Indications: Temporary and immediate relief of pain associated with bursitis, fasciitis, and tendinitis, as well as dispersion of pressure around bone prominences.

Contraindications: Allergies to tape or adhesives, diabetes, or peripheral vascular disease.

Procedure: The general rules for applying tape or adhesives to the skin also apply to the feet. The skin should be healthy, well hydrated, and noninfected. Hair overlying the area should not be shaved so as to avoid irritation and folliculitis. The use of a prewrap prior to taping eliminates the need for shaving and pretape sprays. The materials generally used for padding are adhesive felt or foam of one-quarter-inch or one-eighth-inch thickness,

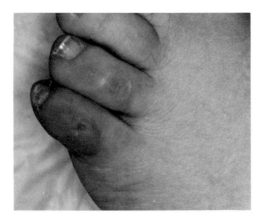

FIGURE 1. Heloma (corn)—discrete area of hyperkeratosis with a central core.

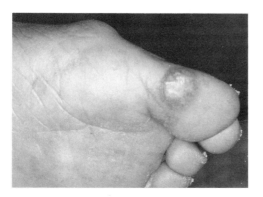

FIGURE 2. Tyloma (callus)—diffuse area of hyperkeratosis.

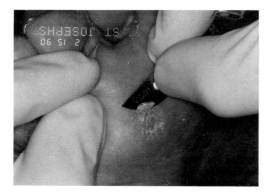

FIGURE 3. Paring of tyloma: The scalpel blade is held firmly between the thumb and index finger and is positioned almost parallel to the callus.

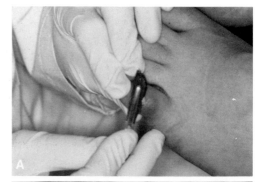

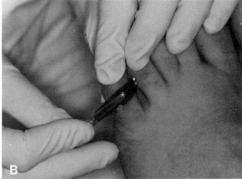

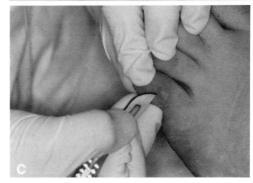

FIGURE 4. *A* and *B*, Debridement of heloma—backhand stroke. *C*, Removal of central core of heloma.

moleskin, roll foam, and tape. Most pads come prefabricated from the suppliers and have adhesive backing.

Bunion pads are fashioned with thicker felt materials. A U-shaped or donut-shaped pad is placed over the dorsomedial bump. The pad is then covered with two or three strips of tape to hold it in place for 2–4 days. Another method is shown in Figure 5. Roll foam is fashioned to cover the hallux and the dorsomedial eminence. The lesser digits are another common area for padding. A smaller U or donut pad is placed over the corn (Fig. 6). These are secured in place by tape or small digital covers (Fig. 7). The digit should never be circumscribed with tape or digital covers, since it can cause constriction and

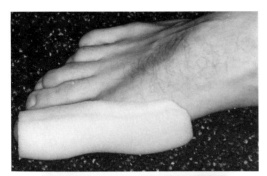

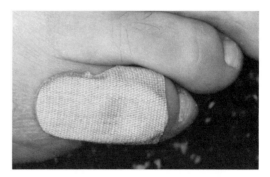

FIGURE 7. Covering over digital padding.

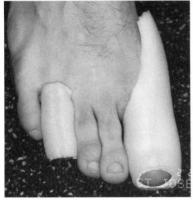

FIGURE 5. Roll foam bunion pad.

circulatory impairment. Roll foam can be used on digits also for dispersion. Lamb's wool, also called angel hair, can be wrapped around the affected digit for temporary relief. The advantage here is that the patient can repeat the procedure daily and there are no adhesives. Temporary relief of submetatarsal pain can be offered by padding. Figure 8 shows a one-quarter-inch thick felt pad placed proximal to the metatarsal heads, which disperses pressure from any or all of the metatarsal heads.

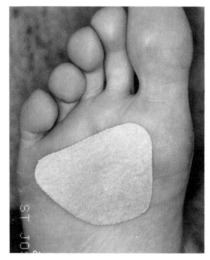

FIGURE 8. Submetatarsal padding with ¼" felt. The pad is placed proximal to the metatarsal heads.

The padding is usually covered with strips of two-inch tape. Moleskin padding is applied directly over the metatarsal heads (Fig. 9).

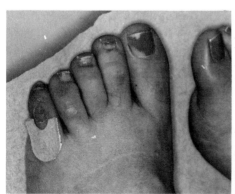

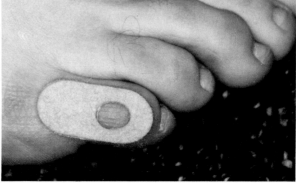

FIGURE 6. Digital corn pad.

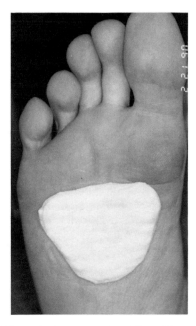

FIGURE 9.   Submetatarsal padding with moleskin. The moleskin pad is placed at the level of the metatarsal heads.

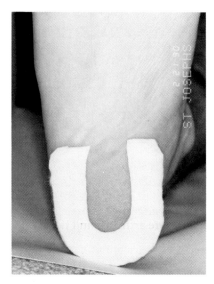

FIGURE 10.   Heel spur padding.

Friction burning and diffuse callus are relieved with a moleskin pad. The pain of **heel spurs** and **plantar fasciitis** can be temporarily relieved by padding or strapping. The heel spur pad (Fig. 10) is made of thicker felt padding and fashioned in the shape of a U. It is applied directly to the affected heel and is covered

with two or three strips of two-inch tape. This pad is designed to disperse weight from the central and more painful part of the heel. For relief of plantar fasciitis, a pad made of one-quarter-inch felt is fashioned to fit the longitudinal arch (Fig. 11A). It is then covered with two-inch adhesive tape, which relieves symptoms by taking tension off the plantar fascia (Fig. 11B). Combinations of these pads can also be used.

Outcome/Prognosis: The patient is instructed to leave the pads on for 1–3 days. If

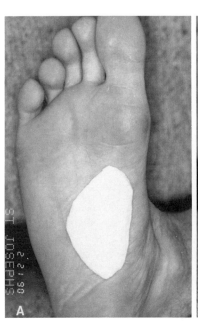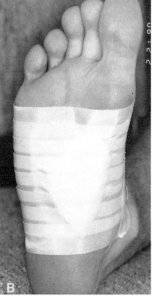

FIGURE 11. *A,* Long arch pad for relief of plantar fasciitis. *B,* One-inch tape covering over long arch pad.

the pads become wet (e.g., from bathing), they should be removed to avoid skin maceration. Padding is generally used as an adjunct to other treatment modalities (i.e., paring, injections, nonsteroidal anti-inflammatory drugs [NSAIDs]); relief lasts for 6-8 weeks. Used alone, relief will last only 3-5 days.

TOENAIL DEBRIDEMENT

Indications: Relief from pain and pressure caused by toenail growth and hypertrophy, especially in patients with diabetes, sight impairment, severe arthritis, and peripheral vascular disease.

Contraindications: Severe diabetes or peripheral vascular disease.

Technique: Proper treatment of the toenails involves cutting the nail straight across (Fig. 12) and maintaining a clean nail groove. The nail grooves are on the medial and lateral borders of the nail, and they extend from the base of the nail to the distal end of the toe. Cutting the nail too short or angling the distal end of the nail causes the distal nail groove to close or narrow. Excessively tight socks or stockings may compress the distal tuft of the toe, pushing the skin proximally and flattening it up against the nail. When the nail grows out, it will be forced to grow into the skin, causing ingrown or infected ingrown toenails. Figure 13 shows the proper technique of debridement of the toenail. The nail splitter used here is held parallel to the distal edge of the nail and perpendicular to the toe. Once this is completed, the nail grooves must be cleaned with a nail curette (Fig. 14). The curette has a cutting edge, so care must be taken not to cut the skin.

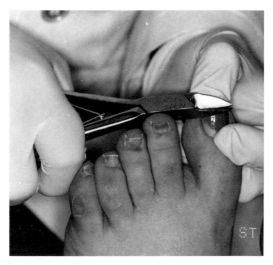

FIGURE 13. Proper technique for toenail debridement.

Outcome/Prognosis: Proper nail care ensures against ingrown or infected ingrown toenails. Treatment should be repeated every 6-8 weeks.

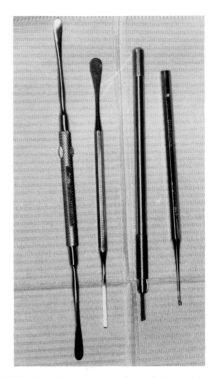

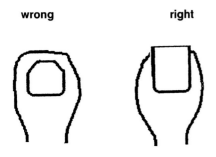

FIGURE 12. The proper way to cut the toenail is straight across. The left drawing shows a short, angled toenail.

FIGURE 14. Instruments (from left to right): nail curette, Beaver No. 61 blade and handle, spatula packer, elevator.

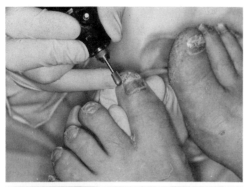

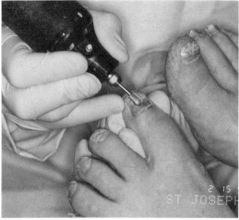

FIGURE 15.   Technique for burring toenails.

ELECTRIC BURRING/ GRINDING

Indications: Smoothing the rough edges of debrided nails and reducing thick nails caused by trauma or fungus.

Contraindications: Hypersensitivity and infected toenails.

Procedure/Technique: After much of the toenail has been debrided with a clipper, the remaining debridement is accomplished with an electric burr. Figure 15 shows the technique of burring a toenail. The dominant hand firmly holds the drill, bracing against the foot with the fourth or fifth finger. The other hand holds the digit from the plantar aspect. The burr is moved from medial to lateral or vice versa, repeatedly until the desired amount of nail is removed. Burring generates heat, so the burr must not be held in one area for long periods.

Outcome/Prognosis: This technique provides 6–8 weeks of relief and should be repeated after that time.

LASER WAFFLING

Indication: Conservative method of curing fungal toenails.

Contraindications: Diabetes or peripheral vascular disease.

Procedure/Technique: A CO_2 laser burns numerous small holes into the affected nail. The laser beam is set so it will not completely penetrate the toenail and cause damage or burns to the underlying soft tissue. Topical antifungal medications are then applied daily by the patient (see Table 1, p. 30). Topical medications used alone do not work well on fungal nails because they are unable to penetrate the thick nail. Laser waffling allows better penetration of these medications.

Outcome/Prognosis: The waffling technique is repeated every 2 weeks. The fungal toenail is cured in 4–6 months if the patient is compliant.

NAIL SURGERY

Indications: Temporary or permanent removal of either the entire nail or part of the nail.

Contraindications: Diabetes, peripheral vascular disease, or bleeding disorders.

Procedure/Technique: After local anesthesia has been administered and the foot and lesion have been scrubbed carefully with povidone-iodine (Betadine) or hexylresorcinol (pHisoHex) solution, the necessary amount of nail is removed. Total nail removal is illustrated in Figure 16. By use of an elevator, the proximal nail fold is freed. Once it is completely free, the elevator is reversed and slipped under the proximal edge of the nail. The nail is then lifted up and off by using the elevator as a lever. The nail matrix, now exposed, can be cauterized or destroyed by either phenol, laser, or surgery for permanent removal if so desired. The technique for partial nail removal is shown in Figure 17. After local anesthesia has been administered and a rubber tourniquet applied, a spatula packer is used to free the proximal nail fold on the affected side. (Note that the tourniquet can also be used in the total nail procedure. A tourniquet should not be used in the elderly or in patients with diabetes or poor circulation.) A nail splitter or an English anvil splitter (Fig. 18) is then inserted and positioned to remove the desired amount of nail. Once this is complete, a hemostat is used to grab the freed nail and remove it.

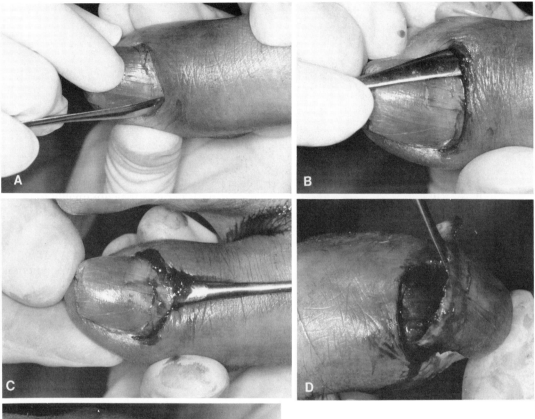

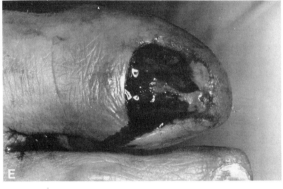

FIGURE 16. *A* and *B*, Total nail avulsion. Nail fold is freed with spatula packer. *C*, Spatula packer/elevator is slipped under proximal nail. *D*, Packer is used as a lever to lift nail from bed. *E*, Nail is completely avulsed.

Excessive granulation tissue can be further removed by trimming with scissors or cauterization with a silver nitrate stick. The nail matrix, now exposed, can be either destroyed by cauterization with phenol or laser or surgically excised for permanent removal, if so desired.

Eighty-eight percent phenol is administered with sterile applicator sticks (Fig. 19). The applicator is dipped in phenol and the phenol applied to the exposed nail matrix for 1–2 minutes. Care must be taken not to get any phenol on surrounding skin. After the applicator is removed, the area is flushed with alcohol to neutralize any remaining phenol.

The phenolized area should turn a grayish white; if this color is not observed, the procedure should be repeated. Range of total application varies from 90 seconds to 5 minutes.

The latest technique is laser cautery of the exposed nail matrix. Figure 20 shows the positioning of the laser beam. The procedure is technically more difficult than the phenol procedure; it requires a steady hand. Once completely cauterized with laser, the exposed tissue turns a brownish-white color; the procedure should be repeated until this point is reached.

Surgical matricectomy is often preferred for young, healthy patients and is accomplished by subcutaneous dissection of the nail

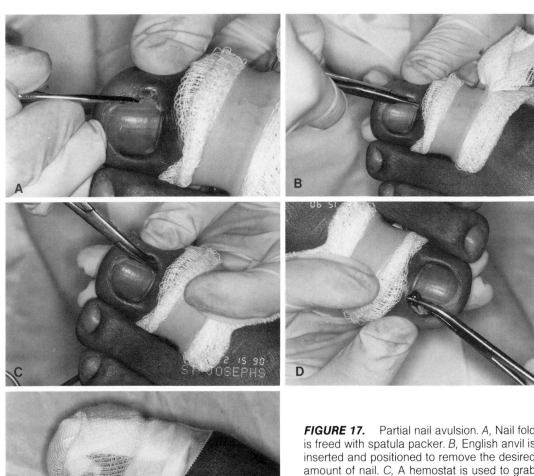

FIGURE 17.   Partial nail avulsion. *A,* Nail fold is freed with spatula packer. *B,* English anvil is inserted and positioned to remove the desired amount of nail. *C,* A hemostat is used to grab the freed nail. *D,* Freed nail is removed. *E,* Bandage after nail surgery.

bed underlying the excised portion of nail from proximal to distal using a No. 15 blade. Matrix fragments are removed with a rongeur, and soft tissue remnants with a Buck bone curette. Excessive tissue voids should be closed with sutures.

Outcome/Prognosis: For nail removal, partial or total, without destruction of the nail matrix, the recovery period is 2 or 3 weeks. An aseptic dressing should be worn until the wound is dry. It is very important to make certain that the toe box of the shoe is adequate. It may be necessary to prohibit both weight bearing and the wearing of a shoe for several days. Modification of the current shoe may be required. The nail will grow back in 3–6 months. The phenol technique for matrix destruction works well but has some drawbacks. The wounds drain for weeks, and there is associated pain. Also, phenol accidentally applied to surrounding skin causes painful burns and skin slough. The laser technique, if not done properly, is associated with a higher incidence of recurrence, although there is minimal drainage and little pain. The postoperative course is much better for the patient with laser. Surgical matricectomies are generally painful. Suture removal takes place 10–14 days depending on wound condition. The recovery period for nail surgery is 4–6 weeks, with

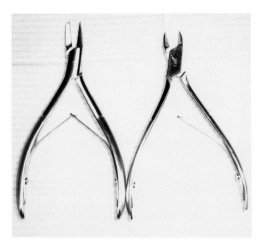

FIGURE 18. English anvil (*left*) and nail splitter (*right*).

evaluation in 4–6 months for nail regrowth. There is a 3–5% incidence of regrowth of nail spicules and/or portions of ingrown nail with chemocautery; surgical matricectomy has a 1% recurrence or regrowth rate. Postoperative analgesics may be necessary.

STRAPPING

Indications: Mild sprains, tendinitis, fasciitis, improvement of foot function, and prophylaxis prior to athletic activities.

Contraindications: Allergy to tape or adhesives, severe sprains, fractures, or dislocations.

Procedure/Technique: The plantar rest strap is used to relieve the symptoms of fasciitis. It is applied by first measuring the amount of one-inch tape needed and applying the end of the *nonadherent side* against the

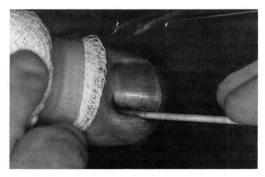

FIGURE 19. Application of 88% phenol to cauterize nail matrix.

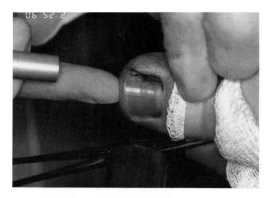

FIGURE 20. Laser cautery of nail matrix.

skin overlying the head of the first metatarsal. The tape is extended proximally around the heel along the lateral aspect of the foot to the head of the fifth metatarsal. At this point the tape is torn and stuck onto the examination table so that it can hang freely. Two more pieces the exact length are measured. Then, using two-inch tape and the same method of measuring, four pieces of tape are measured from the medial aspect of the metatarsal plantarly to the lateral. This tape is placed nearby. Using the one-inch strips, beginning medially at the first metatarsal head, the tape is applied all the way around the foot to the head of the fifth metatarsal. A second one-inch strip is applied on top of the first, overlapping one quarter inch plantarly. The tape should be bowstrung in the arch area. The two-inch tape is then applied from medial to lateral, starting just proximal to the metatarsal heads. The two-inch tape should be based on both sides of the one-inch tape from medial to lateral, and overlapping by one-half inch from distal to proximal. Once all the two-inch tape is in place, the final piece of one-inch tape is applied, as a binder, exactly over the first two pieces of one-inch tape. This strapping will last 3–5 days if it does not get wet.

The **J strap** is a common strapping used by practitioners and athletic trainers to stabilize the subtalar joint and limit inversion or eversion (Fig. 21). It is applied as follows: after prewrap has been applied to the foot and leg, two-inch tape is measured out from the inferior aspect of the medial malleolus to the middle of the lateral aspect of the leg. Three pieces of tape this length are necessary. The patient sits on the examining table with the affected foot hanging off the side. To prevent subtalar inversion, with the foot perpendicular to the leg, the patient everts the foot and holds

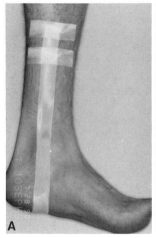
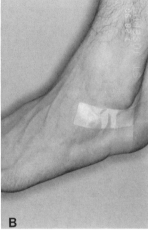
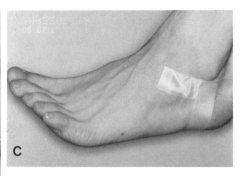

FIGURE 21. J strap. *A,* Boundaries extend from the middle of the medial aspect of the leg. *B,* Extends from the lateral side of the foot just inferior to the lateral malleolus. *C,* View of lateral malleolus and adhesive strap boundary.

it in this position. (If the patient is unable to do this, an assistant can hold the foot in position.) The tape is applied just inferior to the medial malleolus around the plantar aspect of the heel and up the lateral side of the leg. This is repeated with the second and third strips of two-inch tape. Binders are placed across the anterior aspect of the leg where the tape is bow strung, using one-inch tape. (The binders should not circumscribe the leg.) This strapping is reversed to prevent subtalar eversion. It can also be done on both sides, termed the double J, to limit subtalar motion completely.

The **Louisiana heel lock** is used to prevent the symptoms of excessive pronation, ankle sprains and strains, and shin splints (Fig. 22). The anterior of the ankle and both malleoli are protected by the use of Webril or gauze. The wrap starts with one-inch tape on the dorsal lateral surface of the ankle. The tape is rolled around the foot under the arch toward the lateral and proximal aspect on the plantar heel. The tape is then brought up, hooking the lateral side of the heel, and is directed superiorly, posterior to the ankle. Then it runs on the posterior aspect of the calcaneus or over the Achilles insertion headed medially. It crosses over the medial malleolus and ends by crossing over the starting point. With the second piece of tape, the procedure is performed in the opposite direction for the medial heel lock. Strips of one-inch tape are used as anchors over any free edges.

The **Gibney ankle strap/basket weave** allows dorsiflexion and plantarflexion of the ankle, and it limits inversion and eversion of the subtalar joint (Fig. 23). The calcaneus should be placed parallel to the ground and the foot perpendicular to the leg. The first strip of one-inch tape is started on the medial aspect of the leg close to the Achilles tendon, about 5 inches above the medial malleolus. The tape is carried down the leg, under the heel, and up the lateral border of the leg to the same height as the medial side. The second strip is started just proximal to the first metatarsal head, follows the medial border of the foot around the heel, and is ended proximal to the head of the fifth metatarsal. The third and subsequent perpendicular strips are placed parallel to and overlapping the previous strips around one-quarter inch. The fourth and subsequent horizontal strips are placed parallel to and overlapping the previous strips by one-quarter inch. The size of the ankle determines the number of strips used.

INJECTION THERAPY

Indications: Any area where pain and inflammation are localized, that is, not relieved by NSAIDs and conservative physical therapy (e.g., capsulitis, arthritis, bursitis, sesamoiditis, and, most commonly, heel spur syndrome).

Contraindications: Diabetes, peripheral vascular disease, overlying infections, fractures, and known allergies to injectable solutions.

Procedure/Technique: By use of an 18-gauge drawing needle on a 3-ml syringe, 2 ml of a 50-50 mixture of 1% lidocaine hydrochloride plain and .5% bupivacaine hydrochloride plain is drawn. A small amount of a long-acting steroid is then added (e.g., dexamethasone 0.8–1 mg). The area to be injected is surgically prepared with povidone-iodine

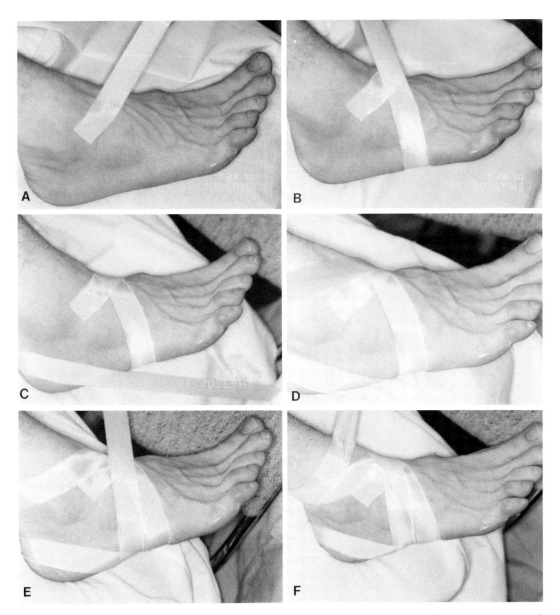

FIGURE 22. *A,* Wrap starts with 1" tape on the dorsal lateral surface of the foot. *B,* Ankle lock: tape rolls around the foot, under the arch onto the lateral side. *C,* Wrap continues over the dorsum, around the ankle, across the heel below the Achilles insertion. *D,* Tape continues across the lateral heel and across the plantar surface. *E,* Tape continues dorsally. *F,* Wrap now covers the dorsum, goes around the ankle covering both malleoli, and ends after the medial malleolus.

and numbed with ethylchloride spray. A 25-gauge 1¼-inch needle is used, and the syringe is thoroughly mixed. The area of tenderness is determined by palpation prior to injection (e.g., medial tubercle of calcaneus for heel spur). The injection should be directed at the area of most tenderness. With a dartlike motion, the needle is advanced, and the area aspirated and infiltrated with the mixture. Tendons should

never be injected. To ensure that the sheath or peritendinous tissue is being infiltrated, the patient should move the muscle tendon unit. Movement of the syringe indicates that the needle is in the tendon. After withdrawal of the needle, the area should be massaged slightly to ensure dispersion of the agents.

Outcome/Prognosis: Relief should last from 1 to 7 days, at which time a subsequent

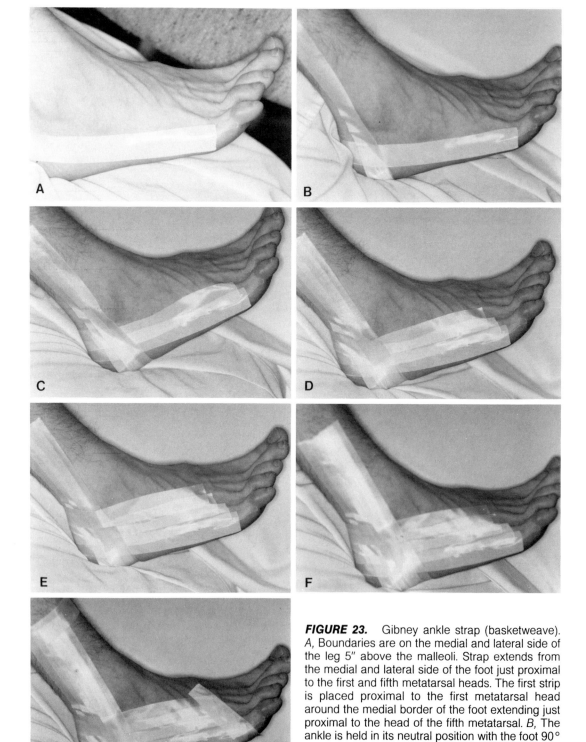

FIGURE 23. Gibney ankle strap (basketweave). *A,* Boundaries are on the medial and lateral side of the leg 5″ above the malleoli. Strap extends from the medial and lateral side of the foot just proximal to the first and fifth metatarsal heads. The first strip is placed proximal to the first metatarsal head around the medial border of the foot extending just proximal to the head of the fifth metatarsal. *B,* The ankle is held in its neutral position with the foot 90° to the leg or slightly plantarflexed. *C,* The process is repeated with ¼″ overlap. *D,* Process repeated with ¼″ overlap. *E,* Process repeated with ¼″ overlap. *F,* Process repeated. *G,* Process repeated.

injection may be necessary. If the pain is not relieved by four injections, surgery should be considered.

ORTHOTICS

Indications: Reduce impact, cushion the foot, relieve pressure and pain, and correct biomechanical abnormalities.

Contraindications: No significant contraindications. Rigid materials should be avoided in patients with diabetes and peripheral vascular disease.

Procedure/Technique: An extensive biomechanical evaluation must be completed prior to casting for these devices (see Chapter 2). Functional orthotics are rigid or semirigid and generally extend up to the metatarsal heads. They are used to correct biomechanical abnormalities. The accommodative orthotic is made to disperse pressure or "accommodate" bony prominences on the plantar aspect of the foot (e.g., plantar corns, heel spurs). These orthotics are made of softer materials such as leather or Plastazote, and can extend to the sulcus or to the tip of the toes. Although accommodative orthotics wear out relatively quickly, they offer the patient months of relief (Table 1). The casting technique that will be described for a foot orthotic appears simple, but unless the foot is positioned exactly right, the results will be unacceptable. Any hyperkeratotic lesions are marked prior to the application of plaster. A cotton-tipped applicator and povidone-iodine solution work well as a marker. The casting takes from 30 to 45 minutes and is performed as follows. The patient lies prone on the examining table with both feet hanging over the edge. Neutral position of the subtalar joint is determined. With one hand holding the fourth and fifth metatarsal heads, the subtalar joint is supinated and pronated repeatedly. The other hand feels for the talar head and positions the foot exactly in neutral. Once the neutral position is found, the patient is asked to hold that position. A five-inch-wide plaster splint precut to the length of the patient's foot is then dipped in cool water, wrung out, and applied to the medial side of the foot from distal to proximal. The plaster splint should not extend to the dorsum of the foot. The plaster is rubbed in thoroughly so it conforms well to the foot. A second splint is then applied to the lateral side in the same manner, again working the plaster in well. Once the plaster has dried, the

TABLE 1. *Orthoses*

General Type	Indications
Soft	
Spenco®	Elderly patients with metatar-
Steinmold®	salgia beyond the age of
PPT®	surgical correction
Sorbothane	Determine whether permanent
(no cast	orthoses are needed
needed)	Pain from overuse injuries
Semirigid	
(neutral cast	Athletes
needed)	Unidirectional sports
	Multidirectional sports
	Skiing
	Control of abnormal prona-
	tion and supination
	Decrease overuse and/or
	acute injuries associated with
	abnormal foot positioning
Rigid	
Rohadur®	Everyday activity (e.g., walking)
	Edge-control sports
	In high-heeled shoes to decrease
	shock of contact at heel strike

slipper cast is then removed. (Shaking the foot or having the patient wiggle the toes makes removal easier. Application of petroleum jelly to the foot prior to casting may also aid in removal.) This procedure is then repeated for the other foot. The cast impressions of the feet are called the negative cast. A positive cast is made from this negative, which will serve as the template for the fabrication of the orthotic. The casts are sent to an orthotics laboratory for fabrication of the specified orthotic.

Outcome/Prognosis: The treatment of pathomechanics is a difficult and challenging endeavor. Functional devices limit pathologic pronation at the subtalar joint, realigning the foot in relation to the supporting surface and reestablishing a normal propulsive sequence. Accommodative devices increase the weight-bearing surface of the foot by bringing the supportive surface up to the foot. This improves weight distribution and symptomatology without necessarily establishing a propulsive gait. In general, accommodative devices are indicated for the more subluxed and deformed foot.

Efficiency of foot orthoses depends on their shape, fabrication, and composition, which should be devised and prescribed with specific goals for total body mechanics. Problems may arise when the body compensates for the new position induced by the orthotics. Such excessive control problems include iliotibial band syndrome, hip rotator strain, greater trochanteric bursitis, exacerbated low back pain, and plantar fasciitis. Solutions include decreasing the control and prescribing exercises to increase the range of motion of all lower-extremity joints.

The patient should be instructed on the break-in period. Orthotics should be worn 1–2 hours for the first day, 2–3 the second day, and so on, until they can be worn all day. The break-in period is generally 2 weeks. Orthotics may need adjustments by the lab if casting techniques were improper.

SHOE MODIFICATION AND MOLDED SHOES

Indications: Conservative treatment for foot ailments, particularly due to diabetes, arthritis, vascular disease, or chronic ulceration.

Contraindications: Fractures, dislocations, or other traumatic injuries.

Procedure/Technique: Athletic running shoes (i.e., sneakers) are a socially acceptable solution to painful dysfunctional feet. Such shoes with wide soles, medial-lateral stability, good arch support, and heel support prevent pronation. Velcro closures improve the ease of opening and closing. In addition, helpful features include cushioning of the sole, soft tops, and a lower heel. Athletic shoes should be used as part of a comprehensive treatment program (i.e., muscle-strengthening exercises, mechanic support, pain relief, weight loss in the obese, and other physical therapy methods). Modifications can be added inside or outside the shoe. Custom-molded orthotic devices can be inserted into the shoe. Plastazote inserts are used in diabetics and ulcer patients to relieve pressure. The depth inlay shoe or extra-depth shoe allows easy insertion of orthotic devices. For adult shoes, most external modifications come in the form of accommodation. Bunion-last shoes have a modification in the last so as to provide more space for the dorsomedial eminence of the bunion and a higher toe box for hammer toes. For regular-last shoes, shoemakers have a device called a swan, which stretches the shoe leather overlying the painful bunion. Submetatarsal pain can be relieved with a metatarsal bar placed proximal to the metatarsals on the sole of the shoe. Limb length deformities also can be accommodated by additions to the sole and the heel. Custom-molded shoes can be used to accommodate for any painful foot condition.

Prosthetics and braces can also be incorporated when necessary.

Technique for Casting for Molded Shoes

The patient is seated. A foam pad covered with plastic is placed under the foot. Petroleum jelly is applied to the foot. Five-inch-wide plaster splints are applied to the plantar aspect of the foot, extending medially and laterally but not dorsally on the foot, and 1 inch above the posterior aspect of the ankle. The foot is placed in neutral subtalar position and then placed, semi-weight-bearing, on the foam pad. The plaster is allowed to dry. Petroleum jelly is applied to the edge of the plaster. The dorsal plaster is then applied, covering the remaining area of the foot completely. Once the plaster is dry, pencil marks are made from the plantar to the dorsal plaster splints for reference points for realignment later. The cast is then removed and sent to a lab for fabrication.

Outcome/Prognosis: The practitioner should keep in mind that once the shoe is modified, the patient is limited to that shoe for relief. Also, once the condition has resolved, the modified shoe may have to be discarded. Shoe modification and molded shoes provide a good method of relief for the nonsurgical candidate. The average shoe lasts from 8 months to 2 years.

SURGERY: GENERAL GUIDELINES

Foot surgery has become very popular over the past few decades, and elective foot surgery is indicated for painful conditions not relieved by conservative therapy. (It is contraindicated in cases of severe diabetes and peripheral vascular disease.) Two options exist: minimal incision, or closed surgery and open surgery. Both require extensive knowledge of foot pathology and anatomy, and both can be done on an ambulatory basis in either a hospital or office setting.

Minimal incision uses small stab incisions, rotary burrs, and drills to grind and cut bone. The bony structures are never directly visualized in this type of surgery. The practitioner must rely on a knowledge of surface and structural anatomy, as well as extensive examination of the joint, including x-rays. X-rays or fluoroscopic views are often taken intraoperatively to ensure proper positioning of instruments. Osteotomies can be made with specialized burrs. Fixation of the osteotomies is seldom used; bandaging holds the osteotomies in place. The skin incisions require only one or two sutures for closure and create minimal scar formation. Tourniquets are not used in this type of surgery.

In open surgery, incisions are made overlying the deformities, which can range from 3 to 12 cm. Tissues are dissected in layers down to bone. Knowledge of deep anatomic tissues and vessels is mandatory. The bones and joints are directly visualized, and osteotomies are fixated by use of screws, wires, and pins according to AO methods. Closure of wounds requires deep tissue closure in layers as well as skin closure, with numerous sutures. Tourniquets are often used in this type of surgery to afford the surgeon a bloodless field. The postoperative course is similar for both methods, and recovery takes between 8 and 12 weeks.

Prior to any surgical procedure, the patient should be informed of the risks and benefits of the surgery. An example of a standard surgical consent form is included in Appendix 5. It should be read and discussed in detail with the patient and his or her family. The surgery, along with the postoperative course, should also be discussed, because the medical and legal ramifications of operating without informed consent can be very costly.

Sterile technique is paramount in any surgical procedure. All articles used in the operation must be sterile, including gloves, gowns, instruments, sponges, and drapes (Figs. 24, 25, and 26).

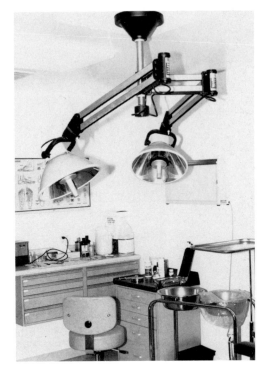

FIGURE 24. Office operating room.

is raised. (To avoid injecting into the extensor tendon, dorsiflexion of the toe will allow the needle to pass underneath the tendon.) The needle is removed completely and anesthesia is injected slowly. The second puncture is made at the site of the medial wheal. Wait for the skin to be numb before injecting. Advance

Local Anesthesia

Once the patient is on the operating table, local anesthesia must be administered. Lidocaine hydrochloride 1% with bupivacaine hydrochloride .5% in a 50-50 mix gives longlasting anesthesia. A hallux digital block is illustrated in Figure 27. Three cubic centimeters of anesthetic solution are injected by a 25-gauge 1¼-inch needle. The initial puncture is made at the base of the proximal phalanx laterally. After aspiration, a wheal is raised at this site. The needle is advanced plantarly, again aspirating and raising a wheal. As the needle is slowly withdrawn, anesthesia is injected. The needle is not removed completely from the first injection site. After aspiration it is advanced to the medial aspect of the digit, where, after aspiration again, another wheal

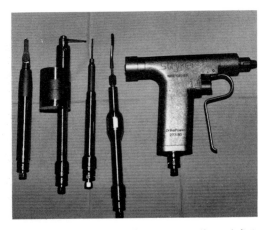

FIGURE 25. Surgical instruments (from left to right): oscillating saw, sagittal saw, drill, reciprocating rasp, wire driver.

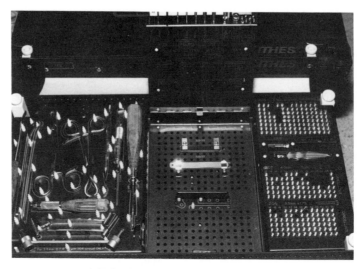

FIGURE 26.   Surgical screw set.

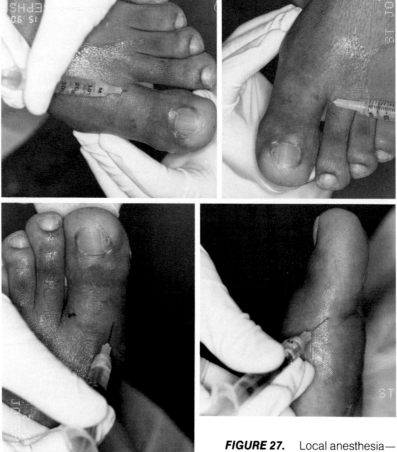

FIGURE 27.   Local anesthesia—hallux block.

the needle plantarly, and aspirate and raise a wheal; injection is made slowly while withdrawing. The third puncture is made at the plantar medial wheal. It is advanced laterally, and the procedure is repeated for the last time. For the lesser digits, the third puncture is not used. Similar technique can be used proximally at the metatarsal level to block for bunion surgery.

Preparation for Surgery

Once the surgical site is numb, it is prepared and draped for surgery. Preparation consists of a 10-minute antiseptic scrub with povidone-iodine. The entire foot should be scrubbed, not just the operative site. Once scrubbing is completed, the foot is dried with a sterile towel and draped. The patient is asked to raise the operative foot, leaving the other foot on the table. The bottom drape is then placed over both the nonoperative foot and the operating table. The operative foot is lowered to the table. A top drape is applied over the patient, exposing only the operative foot. The drape at the patient's head should be raised to screen the operation. After the drapes are in place, the foot is painted with povidone-iodine solution, and the patient is ready for surgery.

Tourniquet

By providing a bloodless field, tourniquets expedite the surgical procedure. For nail surgery, a Penrose drain or heavy elastic band can be used as a tourniquet. It is applied to the proximal aspect of the toe, pulled tight, and clamped with a hemostat. A pneumatic tourniquet is used for more proximal surgery and bone surgery. Applied to the ankle, over some cast padding, the tourniquet is generally inflated to 250 mm Hg. This pressure is tolerable for about 90 minutes. Caution should be taken when procedures last longer.

Suturing

Sutures are used to approximate and hold skin or subcutaneous tissues together until the tissue has enough strength to withstand stress. The technique for simple skin closure utilizes 4-0 nylon on a ½ circle cutting needle. A sterile needle holder, pickup, and scissors are also necessary. For simple sutures, the skin to be sutured is grasped with a pickup (forceps with teeth), everting it. The skin is held with the pickup while the surgeon inserts the needle. The curved needle exerts pressure in the line of the needle, which will allow the needle to slip through the skin easier. In other words, to insert the curved needle, a turning force is exerted on the needle holder. A square knot is tied, and the end of the suture material is cut approximately one-quarter inch. The technique is continued, with sutures spaced evenly, approximately one-quarter inch apart, until the wound is closed. The sutures should remain clean, dry, and intact for 10–14 days.

For suture removal, the area is cleansed with Betadine. The surgeon picks up one of the sutures with a pickup or hemostat and cuts the suture, where is dips beneath the skin, with a scissors or a No. 15 scalpel blade. After it is cut, it is gently pulled out. The process is repeated until all sutures are removed. A sterile dressing is applied to the site for 2–3 days until the suture holes close over.

SURGERY: SPECIFIC PROCEDURES

(The procedures described below are intended to increase the reader's understanding of advanced surgical management of common foot problems. Such techniques are not normally part of the primary care physician's armamentarium, and additional procedural training is required.)

Hammer Toe Procedure/Arthroplasty

As described in the section on corns and calluses, surgery is indicated for permanent correction of painful corns. A standard open-technique arthroplasty will be described. After satisfactory anesthesia, the patient is prepared and draped in the usual manner. A tourniquet is used. Figure 28 outlines two converging semi-elliptical incisions centered over the proximal interphalangeal joint. The incision is deepened, and the skin wedge is removed. Dissection is continued down through the subcutaneous tissue until the tendon overlying the proximal interphalanageal joint is identified. A transverse incision is made in the tendon and capsule at this level. Then all capsular and ligamentous structures are dissected free from the head of the proximal phalanx, and it is delivered dorsally. A double-action bone cutter is then used to resect the

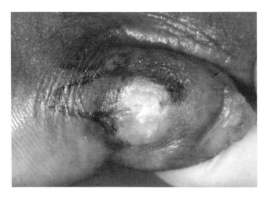

FIGURE 28. Surgical procedure—arthroplasty of fifth toe; skin incision outline.

head of the proximal phalanx (Fig. 29). This is excised in toto. The wound is flushed, the tendon is reapproximated using 3-0 Dexon, and skin closure is made with 4-0 nylon (Fig. 30). The toe is then bandaged with gauze and roll bandages (e.g, Kling). Next,

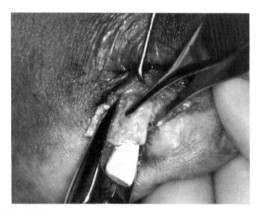

FIGURE 29. Bone cutter resects the head of the proximal phalanx.

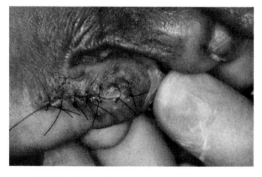

FIGURE 30. Skin closure—arthroplasty.

the tourniquet is released, and capillary return is evaluated to be sure that the bandage is not on too tightly. Postoperative x-rays are taken. The patient is given a postsurgical shoe and allowed to ambulate. The first redressing takes place 3–4 days after surgery. Sutures are removed in 10–14 days, and the patient should be completely out of compression bandages in 3 weeks.

Metatarsal Osetotomy

The indications for a metatarsal osteotomy include submetatarsal bursitis, anterior metatarsal head bursitis, and tailor's bunions. After the osteotomy is made, it is generally fixated with either a screw, pin, or a wire. The procedure for a metatarsal osteotomy for submetatarsal bursitis to the second, third, and fourth metatarsal is as follows: After satisfactory anesthesia, the patient is prepared and draped in the usual sterile manner; a tourniquet is applied to the ankle and inflated to 250 mm Hg. A dorsal skin incision overlying the metatarsophalangeal joint, extending from the base of the proximal phalanx proximally to the distal third of the metatarsal shaft, is made. The incision is then deepened, down through the subcutaneous tissue, taking note of all vital structures. All bleeders are clamped and ligated in the usual manner. Dissection is continued until the extensor tendons are identified and isolated. Retracting these tendons laterally exposes the joint capsule to the metatarsophalangeal joint. A dorsal incision is made in the capsule, and then all remaining capsule and ligamentous structures are dissected free, exposing the surgical neck of the metatarsal. A through-and-through osteotomy from dorsal to plantar is made at this level. The displaced capital fragment is then positioned 1–2 mm dorsal and fixated in place. A 0.045 Kirschner wire is inserted from dorsal proximal to distal plantar. (The wire enters the metatarsal shaft at a 45-degree angle and is advanced into the capital fragment to the level of subchondral bone.) The wire is left protruding through the skin dorsally for easy removal in 3–4 weeks. Deep closure is with 3-0 Dexon, and skin closure is with 4-0 nylon simple sutures. Dry, sterile dressings of 4 × 4 and Kling are applied. The tourniquet is released, and capillary return is evaluated. The postoperative course allows the patient to ambulate in a postoperative shoe. The first redressing is made 3–4 days after surgery. The sutures are removed in 10–14 days. The pin is removed in 3–4 weeks, depending on the x-ray findings.

This procedure can be done by minimal incision as follows: A stab incision is made at the surgical neck of the metatarsal. The incision is deepened down to bone. A periosteal elevator is inserted into the incision to free soft tissue from bone. Once this is completed, a side cutting burr is inserted and a through-and-through osteotomy made at the surgical neck. The skin is then closed with 4-0 nylon. Dry, sterile dressings consisting of 4 × 4 and Kling are applied. The postoperative course allows the patient to ambulate in a postoperative shoe. The first redressing is 3–4 days after surgery. The sutures are removed in 10–14 days. The patient is followed with x-ray evaluations until bone healing is observed.

Fifth Metatarsal Osteotomy

The initial part of the procedure for an open osteotomy is the same as above. Once down to bone, a dorsolateral exostosis will be noted, which must be resected to conform to the normal contours of the shaft. Once this is done, a through-and-through osteotomy is made at the surgical neck. The osteotomy is angled from dorsal distal to proximal plantar and distal lateral to proximal medial. The capital fragment is shifted medially 3–4 mm and dorsally 1–2 mm and fixated in place. A Kirschner wire or monofilament wire can be

used for fixation. For monofilament wire, drill holes are made through the dorsal aspect of the metatarsal to the plantar aspect through the osteotomy. A 2-0 wire is then passed from dorsal to plantar through this hole and tightened onto itself. The wire is cut short and covered over with joint capsule. Deep closure is with 3-0 Dexon, skin closure with 4-0 nylon. Dry, sterile dressing is with 4 × 4 and Kling. The tourniquet is released and capillary return evaluated. The postoperative course is the same as for the other lesser metatarsal osteotomy. There is no pin removal if monofilament wire is used. Preoperative and postoperative radiographs of a bunion and a tailor's bunion are shown in Figure 31.

Bunion Surgery

Bunions are complex surgical procedures requiring extensive knowledge of anatomy, biomechanics, and surgical principles. Four of the more common procedures will be described.

Figure 32 shows a head osteotomy with screw fixation. After satisfactory anesthesia, the patient is prepared and draped in the usual manner. A tourniquet is applied to the ankle and inflated to 250 mm Hg. A skin incision is made, extending from the base of the proximal phalanx proximally to the distal third of the metatarsal shaft. (Figure 32A shows a preoperative foot with four landmark points. Distal is the base of the proximal

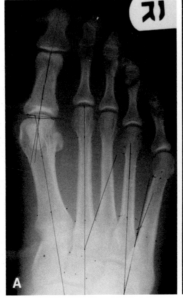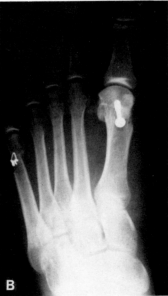

FIGURE 31. Preoperative (A) and postoperative (B) radiographs showing correction of bunion and tailor's bunion.

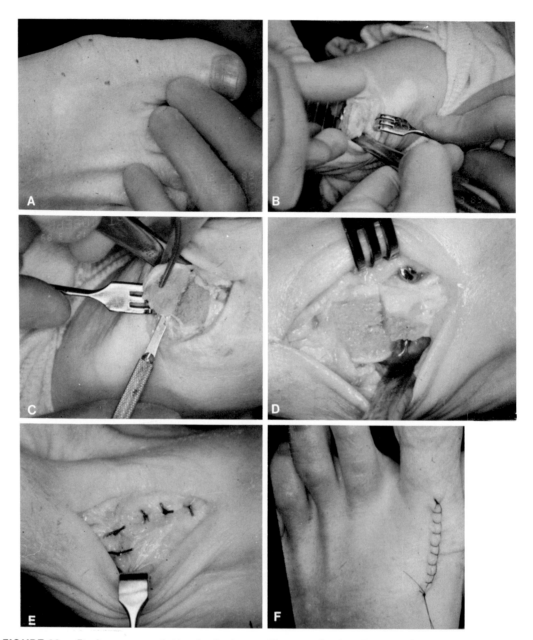

FIGURE 32. Bunion surgery. *A*, Head osteotomy with screw fixation. *B* and *C*, Removal of dorsomedial exostosis. *D*, Osteotomy with screw fixation. *E*, Deep capsule closure. *F*, Skin closure.

phalanx, proximal is the distal third of the metatarsal shaft, medial is the dorsomedial eminence, and lateral is the extensor tendon. The skin incision is from the distal to proximal points, in-between the medial and lateral points.) The incision is deepened through the skin into the subcutaneous tissue. The incision is continued through the subcutaneous tissue, and all vital structures are noted. All bleeders are cut and ligated in the usual manner. Dissection is continued down until the capsule of the first metatarsal phalangeal joint is identified. A dorsomedial linear capsulotomy is then made. All capsular and ligamentous structures are then dissected free from the dorsomedial aspect of the metatarsal head. The dorsomedial bump is resected with an osteotome and mallet to conform to the normal contours of the shaft (Fig. 32B and C). Attention is directed into the first interspace, where, by means of sharp and blunt dissection, the conjoint tendon is identified, isolated, and tenotomized. Returning medially, an L-shaped osteotomy is made at the head. The apex of the osteotomy is midway between the proximal ends of the articular cartilage. The plantar cut is made first and then the dorsal wing. The osteotomy is through and through. The capital fragment is then moved laterally and fixated in place. A Kirschner wire can be used, as described in the lesser metatarsal osteotomy (a 0.062-inch wire is used instead of 0.045). Figure 32D shows the osteotomy with screw fixation. After the osteotomy is fixated, the remaining prominent medial shaft is burred smooth. The area is flushed and closed in layers. Capsule and deep structures are closed with 2-0 and 3-0 Dexon (Fig. 32E). Skin closure is with 4-0 nylon (Fig. 32F). The postoperative course is the same as for the lesser metatarsal osteotomy.

Base Osteotomy

Base osteotomy is used when head osteotomy will not sufficiently lower the intermetatarsal angle. The skin incision is extended proximally to the base of the metatarsal. The procedures done at the metatarsal head are exactly the same as previously described, without the osteotomy. Once attention is directed to the base of the metatarsal, dissection is down through the subcutaneous tissue until the extensor tendons are identified. After they are retracted laterally, the underlying capsule of the metatarsal cuneiform joint is exposed. A dorsal linear incision is made at the base of the metatarsal. The periosteum and capsule in this area are reflected with a periosteal elevator. A wedge osteotomy is then made 1.5 cm distal to the metatarsal base. The apex of the wedge is medial, and the base is lateral. This is not a through-and-through osteotomy; only the lateral cortex is cut completely. The medial cortex must be left intact. A wedge of bone is then removed from this site, again not breaking through the medial cortex. (The amount of bone to be removed is determined preoperatively on weight-bearing radiographs.) The osteotomy is then closed down and fixated with either a screw or a Kirschner wire. The deep closure and skin closure are the same as above. The postoperative course has the patient off weight bearing in a below-knee cast for 4–6 weeks. A longer course of

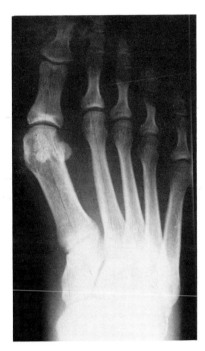

FIGURE 33. Preoperative x-ray of bunion deformity needing base osteotomy.

postoperative physical therapy may also be necessary. Figure 33 shows a preoperative x-ray of a bunion needing a closing base wedge osteotomy. Figures 34 and 35 show two different methods of fixation for the base wedge.

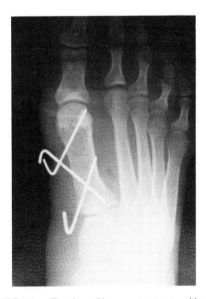

FIGURE 34. Fixation of base osteotomy with cross K wire. Head osteotomy of metatarsal, also fixated with K wire.

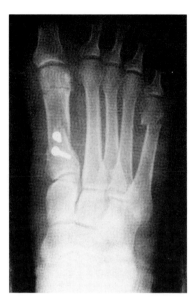

FIGURE 35. Fixation of base osteotomy with screws.

Keller Procedure

The Keller procedure is a joint destructive procedure wherein the distal part of the first metatarsophalangeal joint is removed. Therefore, this procedure is reserved for severely arthritic joints with no possibility of normal function. The procedure starts off the same as the head osteotomy. Once down to capsule, the capsular incision is extended distally onto the base of the proximal phalanx. All capsule and ligamentous structures are then dissected free from the base of the proximal phalanx and the dorsomedial aspect of the metatarsal shaft. The dorsomedial bump is removed with an osteotome and mallet. Attention is then directed to the base of the proximal phalanx, where the proximal one third of the phalanx is resected and excised in toto. The area is flushed and closed as above. The postoperative course allows the patient to ambulate in a postoperative shoe. The first redressing is in 3–4 days, and sutures are removed in 10–14 days. The patient is completely recovered in 4–6 weeks in general. Figure 36 shows the before and after of the Keller procedure. (A head osteotomy was also performed.)

Keller with Implant

Total joint implants are used to restore joint motion (i.e., hallux limitus) and to decrease shortening of the hallux caused by the Keller procedure. The procedure is the same as the Keller, with the following additions: the articular cartilage of the head of the metatarsal is resected perpendicular to the shaft. Once this is completed, the medullary canal of the metatarsal and the remaining proximal phalanx are reamed to accommodate the implant. (Special reamers are available for this

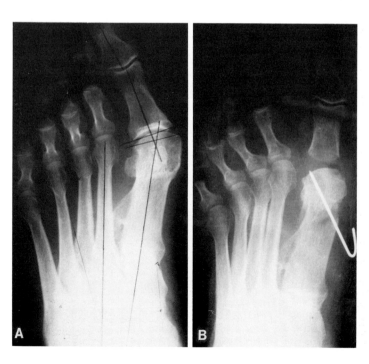

FIGURE 36. Preoperative (A) and postoperative (B) radiographs of Keller procedure with head osteotomy.

procedure.) After that, the implant is inserted, and the overlying structures are closed. The postoperative course is the same as for the Keller. Implants can be used in any of the distal joints of the foot (Fig. 37). Figure 38 shows the before and after of implant surgery.

REHABILITATION AND PHYSICAL THERAPY

The golden period consists of the first 30–60 minutes following trauma. During this period there is much pathologic and histochemical activity (biochemical mediators of inflammation, chemotaxis, vascular permeability, etc.) but relatively minimal or no clinical findings. The treatment for all stabilized trauma is RICE. The R represents rest, which is a relative term (i.e., the injured component is rested, whereas noninjured areas can still be trained). I stands for ice and immobilization. C is for compression, and E represents elevation. This time-honored formula is a simple, cost-effective technique for minimizing the inflammatory response and maximizing functional return.

For the treatment of pain, swelling, and muscle spasm of the lower extremity, long-term use of NSAIDs or oral narcotics is

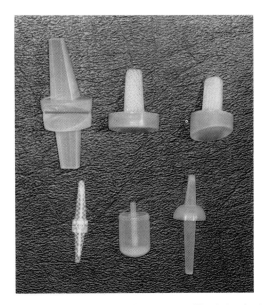

FIGURE 37. Various implants utilized in foot surgery.

contraindicated. Physical therapy modalities constitute an excellent method of treating chronic and acute foot pain with few negative effects. The advantages of using physical therapy alone or as an adjunct to oral or injected medications are the following:

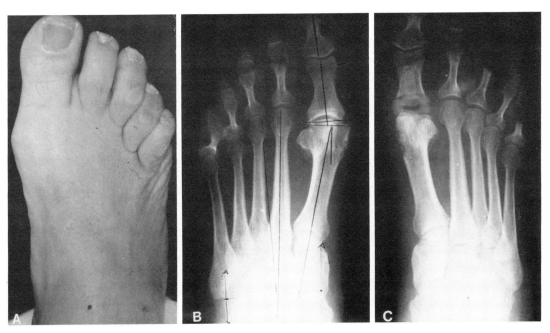

FIGURE 38. Implant surgery. *A*, Clinical appearance of foot. *B*, Preoperative x-ray. (Note the arthritic first metatarsophalangeal joint and osteophytes.) *C*, Postoperative x-ray.

Continued on next page.

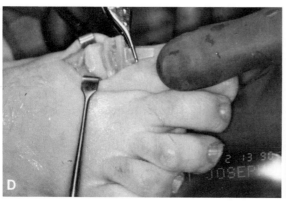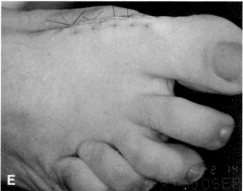

FIGURE 38 *(Cont.).*   *D,* Insertion of the total implant into the first metatarsophalangeal joint. *E,* Skin closure after total joint implant.

1. Local treatment to the affected area.

2. Noninvasive or systemic approach, therefore not causing stomach upset or allergic reactions.

3. Immediate response in acute conditions (e.g., ice for an ankle sprain).

4. Non-habit-forming treatment that can be used as often and as long as necessary.

The objective of physical therapy is either to increase or to decrease blood flow to an area. Heat modalities cause the physiologic response of vasodilation. Vasodilation increases blood flow, which increases inflammation and pain. Cold modalities do the exact opposite: they vasoconstrict. Vasoconstriction decreases blood flow, which in turn decreases inflammatory response and edema.

Heat Modalities

Heat modalities work well on subacute and chronic conditions. They should not be used in the acute condition, because they increase the inflammatory response and the pain. The general rule for acute conditions is cold for the first 24-48 hours and then heat. Heat therapy is indicated for pain and swelling due to rheumatoid arthritis, osteoarthritis/traumatic arthritis, myositis, postsurgery/posttrauma, and muscle spasm.

Heat modalities are contraindicated for the following: circulatory impairments, malignancies, ulcerations or any open wounds, pregnancy, sensory impairments (e.g., diabetes, alcoholism), acute conditions, fractures, apophyseal centers, postsurgical areas where metal screws, plates, and wires are left in place, and infections.

Conductive heat is a superficial heat modality that will penetrate to a depth of 1-2 mm after direct application to the skin. Hot packs, paraffin, and hydrotherapy (whirlpool) are some examples of conductive heat. The temperature must be monitored and should never exceed 106-108°F. Most professional whirlpool and paraffin baths have a thermometer or a thermostat for easy monitoring.

Whirlpool baths (Fig. 39) allow the patient to both receive therapy and perform active range-of-motion exercises at the same time. The ankle, subtalar joints, metatarsal phalangeal

FIGURE 39.   Whirlpool bath.

joints, and digits can be rehabilitated by use of hydrotherapy. Treatments are generally given 10–15 minutes, two or three times weekly until symptoms resolve.

Paraffin is another excellent superficial heat modality. The foot is dipped quickly in the paraffin bath five to ten times. A plastic bag is then applied over the foot, and the patient elevates the foot until the wax cools. This procedure can be repeated two times. It relieves symptoms of all the joints in the foot. Treatment occurs twice weekly.

Radiant heat, a type of convection, is another form of superficial heating. There is no contact with the skin; a heat lamp or infrared lamp is used from a distance. Again, careful monitoring of skin temperature is important. Skin thermometers may be used for this purpose. The modality works well on all inflammatory conditions of the feet. The patient should be lying supine with the feet elevated. Treatment should be given twice weekly.

Conversion heating is a deep heat modality. Electric energy is converted to heat in the deeper tissues. The penetration is much greater than conductive or radiant and heat can exceed 5 cm. Ultrasound is the most common form of conversion heat that is applied directly to the skin (Fig. 40). There are two basic settings—continuous and pulse. The continuous mode is used over soft tissue areas, and the ultrasound transducer must be moved constantly. Conduction jelly must be applied to the skin prior to therapy. There is a large buildup of heat with ultrasound, and burns are a complication. The pulse mode allows the ultrasound transducer to be left in one position, making it effective over bony prominences. The pulse mode does not heat the skin but affects only deep tissue. Contraindications for ultrasound include any metal on the skin or in the deep tissues or bone (i.e., screws, wires, and pins); metal absorbs heat faster than body tissues do and therefore may cause unnecessary burns. Ultrasound is excellent for rehabilitation of all parts of the foot. Treatments are given generally 8–10 minutes, two or three times weekly.

Cold Modalities (Cryotherapy)

Cold modalities work well in acute conditions. They are indicated for acute trauma, pain (topical anesthetic), pruritus, the immediate postoperative period, acute spasm and shin splints.

Cold modalities are contraindicated for circulatory disorders, especially vasospastic; sensory impairments (e.g., diabetes, alcoholism); ulcerations; infections; and stiff joint conditions (e.g., arthritis).

Cold modalities are administered by conduction. Either the affected foot is placed in a cool tank of water or an ice pack is applied. The therapy is given for 10–20 minutes continuously at a temperature less than 15°C, alternating with 20–30 minutes of no therapy

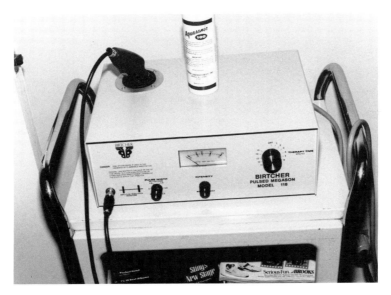

FIGURE 40. Ultrasound unit.

until acute inflammation has subsided. Cryotherapy is best combined with RICE for one acute injury. Cool whirlpools used postsurgically rehabilitate the joint without increasing edema. Treatment is for 10–15 minutes, three times weekly for 2 weeks. Cold therapy is generally a short-term treatment for acute inflammation but may be used in conjunction with heat for a longer term (e.g., contrast bath therapy).

After the acute inflammatory reaction has subsided, range-of-motion (ROM) exercises within the limits of pain are begun. After pain-free ROM is achieved, progressive resistance exercises are started consisting of gradual load increases to an 80-repetition maximum load. These isotonic exercises can be supplemented with isometer (fixed-length) and isokinetic (fixed-speed) exercises.

To rehabilitate the metatarsophalangeal joints and digits, patients try to pick up marbles or a pencil with their toes. Extension and flexion of the digits repeatedly 10–15 times is also effective. To rehabilitate the subtalar joint, inversion and eversion exercises are useful. The patient sits in a chair in front of an open door. With the affected foot alongside the door, the patient is instructed to close and open the door using only the foot. Increased resistance can be placed on the foot by holding the door manually. The exercise is excellent for strengthening chronic ankle instability. To strengthen the ankle joint, the patient should be seated on a high table or chair with the foot dangling. A pocketbook should be hung over the forefoot area. The ankle is then dorsiflexed as much as possible and held for a count of 10 seconds; this is repeated 10–15 times. The exercise strengthens the anterior ankle muscles. To strengthen the posterior muscles of the ankle, heel raises are recommended. The patient stands flatfooted on the floor and raises the heels as far off the ground as possible. He or she may need to hold onto a chair or wall for balance. These exercises should be repeated 10–15 times.

More complex rehabilitative protocols are available and should be handled in conjunction with a physical therapist and physiatrist.

BIBLIOGRAPHY

1. Albom MJ: Avulsion of a nail plate. J Dermatol Surg Oncol 3:34–35, 1977.
2. Albom MJ: Digital block anesthesia. J Dermatol Surg 2:366–367, 1976.
3. Bordelon RL: Orthotics, shoes, and braces. Orthop Clin North Am 20:751–757, 1989.
4. Bunch WH (ed): Atlas of Orthotics, 2nd ed. St. Louis, C.V. Mosby, 1985, pp 346–357.
5. Marshall P: The rehabilitation of overuse foot injuries in athletes and dancers. Clin Sports Med 77:175–192, 1988.
6. McGlamry ED, Banks AS, Downey MS: Comprehensive Textbook of Foot Surgery. Baltimore, Williams & Wilkins, 1992.
7. Molnar ME: Rehabilitation of the injured ankle. Clin Sports Med 7:193–205, 1988.
8. Subotnick SI: Foot orthoses: An update. Phys Sports Med 11:103–109, 1983.
9. Yale I (ed): Podiatric Medicine, 3rd ed. Baltimore, Williams & Wilkins, 1987.

Appendix 1

THE PODIATRY CABINET

The three critical elements for successful management of office patients are an adjustable examination table, a bright operating light, and an adjustable stool. Though an electrically maneuverable podiatry chair provides the greatest flexibility and acceptability for both patient and physician, a standard office examination table is satisfactory. The majority of foot disorders or diseases can be treated and managed by the sitting or standing physician. The examiner's stool should be mobile, on sturdy rollers, flexible to allow for leg length adjustments, and sufficiently comfortable to provide for prolonged sitting.

Office Supplies that Are Useful in the Management of Common Foot Problems

Item	Quantity	Item	Quantity
Cold sterilization tray and solution	1	Nail clippers, small and large	1 each
Electric burr	1	1% and 2% lidocaine (Xylocaine)	1 each
Scalpel blades Nos. 10, 11, 15, and 20	Several	0.5% bupivacaine (Marcaine)	1
No. 3 or No. 4 Bard-Parker scalpel handle	1	Dressing materials	Several each
Flat-jawed tissue forceps*	1	Adhesive surgical tape ½", 1", and 2"	
Curette excavator with 1.5 and 2.5-mm holes*	1 each	Paper tape (hypoallergenic) ½", 1", and 2"	
Medium-size chisel ¼" and ⅜"	1 each	Cotton balls Gauze 2 × 2, 4 × 4 Roll bandages (Kling) Felt adhesive and non-adhesive ⅛" and ¼" Moleskin Cotton/wool ⅛" and ¼" Rubber, polyurethane foam	
Straight nail splitter (thin)*	1		
Suture material	Several each: 000 Dexon/Vicril 2-0 Monofilament 4-0 Monofilament	Plaster of Paris (fast dry) 2", 3", and 4"	Several rolls each
		Plaster splints 5" wide	Several
Straight surgical scissors	1	Solutions	One bottle each: Povidone-iodine Benzoin tincture Ethyl chloride Phenol
Splinter forceps*	1		

*These surgical instruments can be sterilized in a glass bead apparatus in 5 sec at 232°C or 450°F.

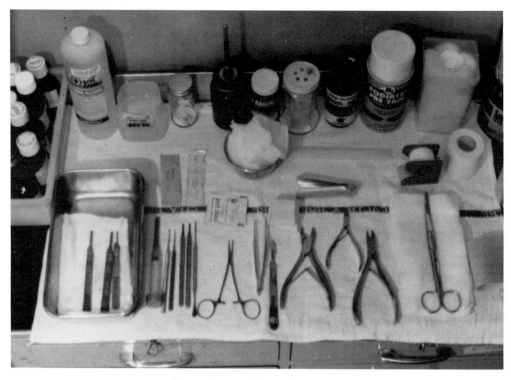

The podiatry cabinet and supplies.

PATIENT EDUCATION MATERIAL
(For Diabetic and Vascular Compromised Patients)

DO

1. Inspect feet daily. Contact the physician at the first sign of redness, swelling, inflammation, infection, prolonged pain, numbness, tingling, or inability to move a foot or a leg.
2. Wash feet daily in lukewarm water (check temperature with hand or elbow) and mild soap; use soft brush.
3. Dry feet by blotting gently, not rubbing, especially between the toes, with a soft towel.
4. Keep feet moist by applying an emollient or lanolin, particularly at the heel margins; use lamb's wool between overriding toes.
5. Use nonmedicated talcum powder or cornstarch if feet sweat easily.
6. Use socks or stockings made from unmercerized cotton or wool that are not wrinkled and are half an inch longer than the longest toe; avoid stretch (nylon) socks, those with an elastic band or garter at the top, and those with internal seams.
7. Beware of new shoes. Choose a shoe according to the following guidelines: soft leather, Blucher type, and a rigid shank or wedge. Or be fitted for a custom-molded shoe, round with high toe box.
8. Break in new shoes slowly and only after they have been approved by the doctor.
9. Inspect shoes daily for foreign bodies such as gravel, protruding nails, torn linings, and the like.
10. Loosen bedclothes to ensure reduced pressure on toes, heals, and bony prominences.
11. Keep feet warm and avoid extreme temperatures.
12. If feet hurt at night, raise head of bed 6-10 inches (15-25 cm) on blocks.

DON'T

1. Use any instruments on the feet.
2. Cut calluses or corns or use chemicals/medications to remove them.
3. Soak the feet.
4. Use hot water, a heating pad, massage, or an electric or mechanic device.
5. Step onto hot surfaces.
6. Go barefoot.
7. Use adhesive tape or other chemicals on the skin.
8. Use inserts or pads without medical advice.
9. Tear or rub nails or skin.
10. Walk in wet shoes.
11. Expose feet to cold weather.
12. Wear sandals or cutout shoes.
13. Wear shoes that are uncomfortable or that rub, blister, or cut into the feet.
14. Cross the legs when sitting.
15. Put cream or lotions between toes.
16. Wear shoes without socks.
17. Use tobacco.

COMMON FOOT TERMINOLOGY

Athlete's foot—tinea pedis, Hong Kong foot.

Ball—area of the foot defined by the widest part of the sole and anatomically consisting of the metatarsal heads and overlying tissue.

Bar (e.g., metatarsal)—a transverse bar consisting of synthetic material (e.g., rubber) across the bottom of the shoe sole with the apex proximal to the metatarsal heads.

Blucher oxford—front-laced shoe pattern with the posterior part of the upper extending just below the malleoli and consisting of a tongue extending from the shoe forepart and tie laces along the sides of the shoe.

Bunion—inflammation of the bursa overlying the metatarsophalangeal joint of the first toe.

Callus—see *tyloma*.

Clubfoot—talipes; types—talipes equinovarus.

Corn—see *heloma*.

Counterreinforcement—a variety of synthetic or natural materials used to preserve the shape of a particular portion of the shoe (e.g., heel counter, lateral or medial counter).

Dancer's foot—inflammatory swelling of the bursa of the first metatarsus associated with high-heeled dancers.

Flare—modification of a last in order to accommodate a natural foot shape or provide correction for an underlying pathology (e.g., in-flares, out-flares).

Golfer's foot—weakness of the anterior arch in association with plantar fasciitis occurring in golfers and other sportsters.

Hallux valgus—deviation of the first toe that becomes curved toward the outer or lateral portion of the foot.

Hammered hallux—dorsal contraction of hallux at the interphalangeal joint.

Hammer toe—dorsal contraction of lesser toe at the proximal interphalangeal joint.

Heel—solid, supporting portion of the posterior shoe, which projects downward (e.g., Cuban, military, flat, spring heel).

Heloma—a localized, inflammatory focus consisting of a core of hyperkeratotic cells composed of impacted, desquamated, dead cells at the site of focal pressure and friction. Helomata may be soft (molle) or hard (durum). Synonym—corn.

Inlay—any type of device that can be inserted into a shoe (e.g., mold, arch support).

Jogger's foot—see *Runner's foot*.

Last—a synthetic or natural model of the weight-bearing aspect of the foot from which a shoe is formed (e.g., straight, combination, bunion lasts).

March foot—fracture of the shaft of the second metatarsal in association with a tender, rounded, dorsal swelling, which may be diffusely cyanotic. The condition was originally described in soldiers, though it is now more commonly seen as stress fractures in runners and joggers.

Pes planus—flatfoot or splay foot.

Runner's foot—medial calcaneal nerve entrapment.

Shank—the area of the last extending from the ball of the foot to the anterior portion of the heel.

Splay foot—a type of flatfoot.

Toe box—area of the shoe forepart that contains the toes.

Toe off—to use the toes to push off during ambulation.

Trench foot—the chronic sympathetic neurovascular changes associated with frostbite that affect the feet of soldiers required to stand for prolonged periods in cold water. Synonym—immersion foot.

Turf toe/toe sprain—the jamming and hyperextending of the hallux into a sneaker.

Tyloma—generalized area of hyperkeratotic skin due to diffuse irritation, friction, or pressure typically at the ball of the foot. Synonym—callus.

SUPPLIERS
OF FOOT PRODUCTS

AliMed
68 Harrison Avenue
Boston, MA 02111
617-451-2240

Apex Foot Health Industries
170 Wesley Street
South Hackensack, NJ 07606
201-487-2739
800-526-2739

Fillauer Orthopaedic
1480 East Third Street
Chattanooga, TN 37401
615-698-8971

Knit-Rite
2020 Grand Avenue
Kansas City, MO 64141
816-221-5200
800-821-3094

Mayflower Podiatry
28 Jericho Turnpike
Jerico, NY 11753
516-333-5400
800-645-3000

Rubatex Corporation
906 Adams Street
Bedford, VA 24523
703-586-2611
800-346-1499

Spenco Medical Corporation
P.O. Box 2501
Waco, TX 76710
817-772-6000
800-877-3626

CONSENT FOR MEDICAL
OR SURGICAL PROCEDURE

PATIENT'S NAME: _____ DATE OF SURGERY: _____

TIME OF SURGERY _____ A.M. _____ P.M.

☐ 1. I, (or_____ for _____) hereby authorize
Dr. _____, and/or such assistants as may be selected to treat
the following condition: _____
_____
_____

(Explain the nature of the conditions and the need to treat such.)

☐ 2. The procedure(s) necessary to treat my condition has (have) been explained to me by
Dr. _____, and I understand the nature of the procedure to
be: _____
_____

(A description of the procedures in layman's language.)

☐ 3. I have been made aware of certain risks and consequences that are associated with the
procedure(s) described in Paragraph 2 such as, but not limited to, *POSTOPERATIVE
INFECTIONS, DELAYED HEALING, NUMBNESS AROUND THE OPERATIVE
SITE(S), POSTOPERATIVE SWELLING, EXCESSIVE AND/OR PAINFUL SCAR
FORMATION, RECURRENCE OF THE PROBLEM.*
Dr. _____ has also explained possible alternative methods of
treatment. I hereby acknowledge that I understand the information given me.

☐ 4. I understand that the explanation of the risks and consequences that I have received
is not exhaustive and that other, more remote risks and consequences may arise. I have
been advised that these more remote risks and consequences will be explained to me
upon request. I acknowledge that I have been given the opportunity to ask questions
concerning this procedure and its risks and consequences, and my questions, if any,
have been answered to my satisfaction.

☐ 5. It has been explained to me that during the course of the procedure, unforeseen conditions may be involved that necessitate an extension of the original procedure(s) or different procedures and that Dr. _____, the assistants, or the designees may perform such surgical or medical procedures as are necessary and desirable in the exercise of their professional judgment. The authority granted under this paragraph (5) shall extend to treating all conditions that require treatment and are not known to Dr. _____ at the time that the operation or procedure is commenced.

☐ 6. I consent both to the administration of anesthesia to be applied by or under the direction of the surgeon, Dr. _____ or the designees and to the use of such anesthesia as they may deem advisable.

☐ 7. I acknowledge that I have received no guarantee concerning the medical or surgical procedure to which I am consenting.

☐ 8. I hereby authorize Dr. _____ either to dispose of any tissues or organs removed as a result of the procedure authorized above or to preserve such tissues or organs, at discretion, for scientific or teaching purposes.

☐ 9. I acknowledge that I have read this document in its entirety, that I fully understand it, and that all blank spaces have been either completed or crossed off prior to my signing.

_____ _____ _____
Witness   Signature of Patient   Date

(If patient is unable to sign or is a minor, complete the following.)

Patient is a minor _____ years of age or is unable to sign because:

_____ _____ _____
Witness   Relative or Legal Guardian   Date

INDEX